TOGETHER, WE WILL
GET YOU BETTER

FUNCTIONAL MEDICINE IN PRIMARY CARE

DR. AUNNA C HERBST

authorHOUSE®

AuthorHouse™
1663 Liberty Drive
Bloomington, IN 47403
www.authorhouse.com
Phone: 1 (800) 839-8640

© 2020 Dr. Aunna C Herbst. All rights reserved.

No part of this book may be reproduced, stored in a retrieval system, or transmitted by any means without the written permission of the author.

Published by AuthorHouse 01/30/2020

ISBN: 978-1-7283-4526-0 (sc)
ISBN: 978-1-7283-4524-6 (hc)
ISBN: 978-1-7283-4525-3 (e)

Library of Congress Control Number: 2020901976

Print information available on the last page.

Any people depicted in stock imagery provided by Getty Images are models, and such images are being used for illustrative purposes only.
Certain stock imagery © Getty Images.

This book is printed on acid-free paper.

Because of the dynamic nature of the Internet, any web addresses or links contained in this book may have changed since publication and may no longer be valid. The views expressed in this work are solely those of the author and do not necessarily reflect the views of the publisher, and the publisher hereby disclaims any responsibility for them.

Doctors, a gift for your patients, and patients, a gift for your doctor

—Dr. Herbst

CONTENTS

Preface ix

Acknowledgments xiii

Introduction xv

Chapter 1   What Is Functional Medicine? And Why? 1

Chapter 2   Lifestyle Modification: Diet, Exercise, and Sauna 20

Chapter 3   CFS: AKA Systemic Exertion Intolerance Disease (SEID) or Myalgic Encephalomyelitis (ME) 32

Chapter 4   Autoimmune Disorders 44

Chapter 5   Thyroid: "The Master Gland" 50

Chapter 6   Vitamin D 59

Chapter 7   Cardiometabolic Health (Hypertension, Cholesterol, Diabetes/Insulin Resistance) 66

Chapter 8   Diabetes/Insulin Resistance 78

Chapter 9   Genetics 83

Chapter 10 Lab Orders: What Will Be Your Biggest Return
on Investment (ROI)? 90

Chapter 11 Case Example: Functional Primary Care 92

Chapter 12 Pediatric Concerns: PANS, PANDAS, and ASD........100

Chapter 13 Tick-Borne Illness, Including Lyme Disease and
Post-Lyme Syndrome 103

A Note from the Author..109

Appendix A—MSQ 111

Appendix B 113

Abstract.. 115

Registered Dieticians 117

Consolidated References... 119

PREFACE

Twenty-two years ago, laying on the floor, sick and exhausted, I promised then to help others. And now I vow to respectfully educate. I hope this book will teach health-care providers who want to be compassionate, understanding healers a way to approach the complexity of individual diagnoses.

My life has led me here. Once a patient, now I am a physician, a doctor with a passion to remind practitioners how to have a happy career and a panel of healthy patients. This book is my gift to all who believe compassion can be mixed with knowledge. Optimal health requires a patient to tell their story and a physician to listen. Restoring optimal function to a body will restore hope in health care!

My goal is to change health care as it stands. Basic changes, which I feel have huge returns, are needed. I was a patient for many years for whom the acute care model did not work. I flailed my way through the health-care system, and out of desperation, I saved my own life, only after I got down to the root of my problems. Later I found out that this is the principal foundation of a new and rapidly growing field of health-care practice called functional medicine.

Before I became a board-certified, family medicine physician and a certified functional medicine practitioner who was one of the pioneers for the prestigious Cleveland Clinic Center for Functional Medicine, I learned that optimizing health is key.

This is the foundation of a systems-based approach to chronic disease, termed *functional medicine*, but functional medicine requires separate, in-depth training, heading back into the first years of medical school, revisiting pathophysiology and biochemistry. Also its approach to patients depends on a substantial amount of office time with the patient, something most of us do not feel we have.

We all want better outcomes for our patients; thus, I am offering a solution for practitioners who have a career in medicine. If you are a clinician helping others with chronic, multisystem-based illness, it matters not whether you practice in the insurance-dominated, time-limited, number-crunching medical model (in which most doctors, physician assistants, and nurse practitioners are required to see patients) or are seeing patients in a cash-concierge practice. I have found several tools that result in better patient-physician relationships and ultimately improved patient health.

The second reason I feel it is time for a book of this kind is because too many of my colleagues are feeling the pressures to see more patients, which means less face-to-face time with patients, yet we are all dealing with increasingly sicker patient populations. After a time, one starts to feel dissatisfied with their career because they do not know how to help some of the most complex cases. Nor do they feel they are stopping disease progression.

Burnout is real, and we cannot afford to have less clinicians available to our nation. And patients need more than a pill to fix their ailments. Patients long to be heard, and they deserve someone who will look for the reason they are ill and help them stop it.

Throughout this book, I will share simple key principles and clinical tools for many topics, including but not limited to autoimmune disorders, genetic polymorphisms and epigenetics, and cardiovascular disease. This will be based on my thousands of successful patient-centered interactions and current supporting literature gathered over the last nineteen years.

I was diagnosed with several ailments: fibromyalgia, chronic fatigue, severe erosive oral lichen planus, and migraines, a true multi-system dysfunction. My full story follows, but for many years, I was desperate for a healing and intuitively knew the diagnoses were not separate etiologies. However, I am sure finding the common cause was integral in my recovery. Lifestyle change and functional medicine is the reason I now stand strong and healthy.

Thus, I am dedicated to optimal health for my patients, and I am passionate about sharing this approach of functional primary care with my fellow health-care providers.

Ultimately it is my desire to help clinicians better serve their patients while at the same time assist in the restoration of the physician's satisfaction in their career choice.

ACKNOWLEDGMENTS

I am thankful for all those who have supported me throughout my journey. I am grateful for all the teachers who have come along and those yet to cross my path. Whether it be a brief interaction or a lifelong walk, I look forward to more such experiences.

Thank you to my family and friends. Without your love and support over the years, there would be no book. Last but not least, thank you, my readers, for without your tenacity and compassion, health care cannot change.

INTRODUCTION

Over the last nineteen years, I have worked as an employee in an insurance-based model and on my own in a cash-based model, and I am here to tell you that there are ways you can utilize true functional medicine without compromising your current work situation.

In this book, I promise to share with you a modality of practice that can look at root cause and optimize function with practical application. With this approach of functional primary care, you will restore your patient's hope, which understandably leads directly to active participation in health and improved patient outcomes and indirectly results in regaining your true sense of self. It has been the experience for myself and others, whom I have counseled in this practice style, that we can get patients better together.

As you traverse through my nine and a half-year health journey to recovery, you will better understand why I practice the way I do. I was implementing functional medicine in pieces, before it was even in existence. Identifying how all my illnesses and diagnoses were similar and interconnected was truly my saving grace.

Now as a board-certified family physician who integrates functional medicine, in a style I termed *functional primary care*, I am pleased to say I am a successful business owner and mother. It's funny how life works. Here is my story.

It all started when I was eight years old. We moved to the country in Oklahoma. I'm talking living in a tent/well house and bathing in the creek kind of country. My father was building a log cabin. And every night's bedtime routine entailed what we called a "tick check," a bathtub soap from head to toe and a dry-off where I'd stand with arms open, like a starfish, while my sweet mother would check to see if we had any embedded ticks. The average was usually three per day.

My sisters and I were very active children, all healthy, breastfed, and without any antibiotics. A well-balanced, yogurt-making, garden-growing family raised us. A few months into us living there in the backwoods, I started to have severe daily headaches, which persisted and became so frequent and routine that I began to count the days, hoping I would be able to enjoy the weekend and planning when I would be able to spend the night with my friends.

Knowing my pattern, I often remember thinking, *Oh good, it's Thursday, so I won't have a headache Friday. I can spend the night with my friend and not have a headache.* Most nights, I would lay in bed, put a pillow over my head, and hold it as tight as I could until I fell asleep. At the same time, I also started having severe abdominal pain, often crying to my mom as I sat on the toilet, cramping with clammy sweats. I had a few bouts of pinworms because, yes, I played in the dirt and was barefoot most of the time.

As for my sleep, my mother says I've always been a light sleeper, even as a baby. However, I recall at that time always waking up around two or three in the morning and laying there awake and waiting for morning to come. I knew it was almost time to get up when I heard the ducks and the geese on the front porch, making their noise below my window.

My parents finally took me to the doctor for my headaches, and he said it was probably because I was "allergic to my stuffed animals." Sadly, this resulted in a purge of my furry-friendly fellows who sat on my shelves and bed. However, we found out it was not the source of my headaches. The constipation and severe abdominal pain were written off as "normal bowel habits with slow transit time." My family was tough. We didn't complain. We didn't go to the doctor so because there was no answer and they were told that "this was normal," we all did our best to ignore my constant symptoms.

As proof my body was in a state of immune dysregulation, I had a few severe cases of strep throat and poison ivy during these two and half years. And so life persisted this way for the next couple years. When I was ten, we moved overseas, and my headaches seemed to dissipate. (We were no longer eating dairy from the farm. [Bummer, no more homemade butter.] We were eating predominately vegetables and fish.)

We were overseas for about six years. We returned to the United States in 1988. About this time, my menstrual cycle started, and the headaches increased in frequency and severity again. At school, I was eating typical American food, AKA the Standard American Diet (SAD), which consisted of dairy, candy, soda, and fried foods.

I continued to be a go-getter, type-A personality with good grades, student council, diving team, and any volunteer activity I could get my hands on.

During high school, my muscle pain became intense, and I seemed to have muscle strains regularly. My sleep continued to be an issue. I didn't sleep as a matter of fact. I found it difficult to fall and stay asleep. But I didn't know any better. I thought this was my new norm—just kept fighting and consuming a lot of aspirin, ibuprofen, and Tylenol. Bowel movements now were once a week.

I went on to college and was very active; however, my migraines continued to increase in intensity, especially significant, after I started on birth control. I really wanted to go to medical school, but I knew with the severe migraines and fatigue I was experiencing, it would not be possible. Despite this, I was physically active, walking many miles a day to class and working out. My diet consisted of "healthy," so I thought, Pop Tarts because they had strawberry filling in them. (Sigh, I knew better, but I was trying to tell myself they were somewhat healthy.) I pushed through as much as I was able.

I wasn't eating anything nearly as healthy as my mother would cook at home. I was now on my own, living on Ramen noodles, canned tuna, microwave popcorn, and the occasional roast and potatoes I would make, along with added frequent treats of ice cream and milkshakes. I would buy apples on occasion and dip them in caramel, thinking this was healthy as well. It's a fruit after all!

I also continued to swim. I was in a chlorinated pool almost daily from the age of fifteen to twenty-one. As a lifeguard and swim instructor, I swam on a swim team and was a springboard diver. This is a possible environmental exposure with negative health effects.[2]

I graduated college and moved to South Carolina. At that time, my identity was that of a no-quitting, I-can-do-anything, confident, take-care-of-others-before-yourself, rest-is-for-the-weak kind of person. I was pushing myself hard, working in the field of research and striving to maintain an image of health, strength, and beauty. I'd end most days with intense physical activity after work, usually riding bikes for hours with my soon-to-be husband. All the while, my body was telling me to slow down. Internally I remember thinking I was exhausted.

Soon after I moved to South Carolina, my appendix nearly ruptured, likely a result of years of constipation, and I ended up in the hospital with emergency surgery. I naïvely thought this would help my bowel movements become more regular. Not!

Eventually I married and soon became pregnant. This was the best I've felt in my entire life. The last two trimesters of my pregnancy were amazing. I slept well, my pain was gone, and I had no migraines. Some speculate this was due to the higher levels of hormones. At the same time, I received news that my Pap smear had returned abnormal.

A well-meaning physician called me into the office and told me that I should terminate the pregnancy, as it was early. I had cancer cells, and the estrogen would likely exacerbate the cancerous growth. I had no idea what they were talking about since I wasn't in medicine at that time, and I was in a bit of shock. I naïvely ignored his advice and continued on with the pregnancy.

I had a beautiful, healthy baby girl. But as soon as I delivered her, my health crashed. Throughout the pregnancy, I had three biopsies taken, and the cancerous cells remained stable after a loop electrosurgical excision procedure (LEEP) procedure.

I was breast-feeding on demand and not sleeping. My hormone fluctuations were drastic, and my migraines were so intense that I was nonfunctional for the most part. My fatigue amplified. I could barely do anything. Then I developed a symptom that was even more inconvenient and devastating, vulvar vestibulitis. The mucosa of my vaginal lining and vulvar area became ulcerated. It was extremely painful to urinate, sex was unbearable, and I was not able to wear pants or open and close my legs without pain. This meant basic everyday activities like walking and urinating were excruciating. My body was falling apart. The muscle pain I felt was intense and persisted for the next two years despite my many visits to specialists. All their recommendations were failing me.

I was also carrying the burden of guilt and failure. I felt guilty, as if I had failed my husband and everyone around me. I was no longer able to participate in physical activities, like bike riding and family hikes. Intimacy and intercourse was incredibly painful, which was discouraging for both of us. Here I was, newly married and a mess. I was becoming desperate. For almost two years, I tried anything and everything the doctors were suggesting. I was feeling as though I was a failure because I wasn't getting better.

Thankfully, my personality did not allow me to give up. My final visit with a renowned specialist for vulvar vestibulitis at the University of Michigan was the straw that broke this camel's back. This doctor had tried everything from medications to hormones and laser removal of the mucous membrane.

And out of frustration, she said, "Maybe you would benefit from an antidepressant." She callously implied this was a mental condition and not a physical one. She handed me a prescription for a tricyclic antidepressant.

I left the office crying and frustrated, though I realize she was partially correct. There was possibly an element of depression but definitely a large bit of hopelessness. After that visit, when my husband picked me up, I kept saying through snots, snorts, and tears, "My vagina is not depressed!"

Admittedly, I did have postpartum depression for twelve weeks after delivery, but not at the time of this appointment. I did not agree with her diagnosis or recommended treatment because once the postpartum depression resolved, all my other symptoms persisted.

There I was, sitting in the car with my kind, young, new spouse looking at me as if I had truly gone mad. When the tears flowed down, my left brain kicked in. I asked my husband to drop me off at the medical library for a few hours, and I started researching.

I scrapped all my diagnoses, like fibromyalgia. (What the heck was that anyway? No one even knew about it. The neurologist who suggested that diagnosis was ahead of his time). I also scrapped vulvar vestibulitis, migraines, IBS, and insomnia. I decided to look for commonalities, overlapping symptoms.

As I sat there, the only thing I knew for sure was I was once healthy and progressively since I was eight years old, my health deteriorated.

Something was wrong, and these diagnoses were a sign of that! This started me on my new journey.

In my hours at the library, I stumbled upon a researcher, Dr. Solomon, from Colorado, who was researching and treating vulvar vestibulitis by using two supplements, calcium citrate and N-acetyl glucosamine, in conjunction with a low-oxalate diet. Following his recommendations, I embarked on a new diet and a few supplements. At the time, surprisingly within about two weeks, I was noticing some improvement in my vaginal pain. This was more improvement than I had had in two years. This was the boost I needed. It was a sliver of hope. Though intercourse remained painful, I used numbing cream, and this resulted in the conception of our second child.

This pregnancy, however, I was very aware of what I was eating. My vaginal pain was improving. However, my fatigue and generalized muscle pain were extreme, except again in the last two trimesters of my pregnancy. By this time, I realized the high levels of progesterone in the latter two thirds of pregnancy was anti-inflammatory, likely part of the reason I felt so well. Later in my studies, I learned it is also very sedating, which is why I was sleeping better.

The answer seemed so simple to me, as I was naïve to the complexities of the endocrine system. I thought I had symptoms of low progesterone; thus, I thought replacing progesterone would be the answer. Like many physicians and patients, I was thinking linear. In other words, I thought I could just take high-dose progesterone after delivery and continue feeling well.

However, after I birthed my second child, my health again deteriorated. I was humbled. The high-dose progesterone prescribed by my OB/GYN did not work. The fatigue and generalized muscle pain were so severe that I recall having to pick and choose my activities during the day. Migraines were frequent. Triptans were not working and easily triggered by fatigue.

At one point, regular activities of daily living were exhausting. If I did more than one household chore, I was guaranteed to be in bed at least for the next twenty-four hours. What had my life become? Lack of sleep and the stress of life was not helping, but there had to be more. I was happy to be a mom, and I looked forward to our family life. I knew this was not postpartum depression. I was happy, but just exhausted.

I was done. I was exhausted and wanted so badly to feel vibrant again. My primary care physician (PCP) decided it was because I was a new mom and the vaginal pain and migraines were hormonal. A neurologist diagnosed it as chronic fatigue, but my PCP remarked that it was not a true diagnosis. I was again confused and alone.

I decided once again to fight. I knew I improved a bit with dietary changes and journaling, so I drastically changed my diet in an attempt to reduce inflammation.[1]

I cut out sugar, dairy, and meat, and I saved my money for a juicer. I began reading more and more, actually copious volumes of books, which led to an online naturopathic course. I knew there was something to this natural approach because slowly I was getting better. All the while, I was persistently seeking the treatment, that is, still linear thinking. It may sound like I was full of energy, but I was very conscious of my energy ... or lack thereof. If I pushed too much, I would land in bed for a day or so to recover with a few days of severe muscle and joint pain.

I was so desperate that I was trying most anything and everything. One of my most diligent focuses was on gut health and nutrient support.

---

[1] A diet high in processed foods, grain-fed meats, and high-sugar foods has shown to be a cause of increased oxidative stress/free radicals.
Bee Ling Tan, Mohd Esa Norhaizan and, and Winnie-Pui-Pui Liew, "Nutrients and Oxidative Stress: Friend or Foe?" *Oxid Med Cell Longev* (2018), doi: 10.1155/2018/9719584.
Frederick D. Provenza,[1*] Scott L. Kronberg,[2] and Pablo Gregorini,[3] "Is Grassfed Meat and Dairy Better for Human and Environmental Health?" *Front Nutr* 6 (2019): 26, doi: 10.3389/fnut.2019.00026.

I found rotational probiotics[2] was best for me. Some of the herbs I consumed were broad-spectrum antimicrobial. So it is very possible that I was stimulating an immune reaction for a possible viral burden. Who knows?

I had no testing done as I was self-treating with nutrition and I found no physician willing to help or listen to my theories. However, I am 100 percent certain, at the end of those months, I made a step in the right direction. I had a marked improvement in my health. Even now, I continue to appreciate the complexity of the human body and its dynamic interaction with our environment.

Ultimately, I believe that juicing turned my health path around for the better. I started juicing from the beginning, right after I had my ultimate breakdown. It is my theory that the readily available vitamins and minerals and enzymes in the vegetable drinks were easily assimilated and absorbed, replacing nutrients my body needed to repair.

We eventually moved to get close to family, and by this time I had studied integrative/alternative medicine for approximately three and a half years, including an online naturopathic certification through Trinity Natural Health College. I understood lifestyle was key. Each time I offered some advice or suggestions for people, I heard the same comment over and over, "You should make this a business." So I did just that: part-time lifestyle counselor and full-time mommy. It was 1999. My health had improved so much that I was ready to give back.

---

[2] Rotational probiotics means consuming different strains by taking one supplement with several strains for two to four weeks and then changing the species for the next two to four weeks and so on.

One of the most significant healing episodes for myself was during this time when I was able to participate in a homeopathic psychology[3] course. I volunteered because I thought I had no emotional baggage. My family life was amazingly well without any trauma and abuse. My left brain, a research-oriented personality, was doubting this whole philosophy of medicine. There I was, pompously sitting in front of a hundred people while a British psychologist asked me, "Of what are you most afraid?"

Humbly, I may not understand the exact mechanism of action of homeopathy; nor am I an expert in this field. But I know in my heart the process I went through that day was incredibly healing. I was afraid of failure. I was afraid of disappointing people I loved. This fear played a huge role in my day-to-day choices, and my internalization of that manifested itself in many ways physically, I believe.

As a result, after many tears and amazing professional support in that room, this too became a part of my healing journey. I realized then that emotional components to disease exist. Over the years as an osteopathic physician, I have often seen this to be the only etiology of a person's presentation.

BY now, it had been four years. I was not 100 percent, but I was sleeping regularly, my bowel movements were getting more regular, and my headaches were only on day one of my menses. I was feeling fantastic! My business flourished. My lifestyle counseling practice was successful. I was able to help my clients change their eating habits and focus on more self-care.

---

[3] Homeopathic psychology philosophy: Symptoms, including psychological ones, are presumed to be ways that the body-mind is trying to adapt to and deal creatively with various internal and external stresses. Psychotherapeutic techniques tend to elicit the patient's symptoms in a controlled manner in order to heal the patient. Such is the case in cognitive, behavioral, and psychoanalytic treatments. In his article, Davidson discusses other points such as the self-healing principle, the micro-dose effect, disappearance of the symptoms in reverse order of their appearance, and diagnosis by pattern recognition of the symptoms (Davidson 1994).

In 2001, I decided I wanted to go to medical school. I sold my business and went to medical school in 2003. This is where my lifestyle training played a huge role. In the following chapters, I will share lifestyle practices I was able to uphold in the four years of medical school that helped me maintain my health. My routine was not limited to but consisted of juicing, sauna, and healthy eating habits.

My journey continued through residency, as I had a pretty significant flare of a rare autoimmune disorder. (I now realize this autoimmune disorder was what presented as vulvar vestibulitis many years before.) The diagnosis in 2009, verified by multiple biopsies, was severe erosive oral lichen planus, a rare immune disorder that attacks mucous membranes, joints, and skin.

2009 was my last year of medical training. I was elected chief resident and working many hours. I had very irregular sleep patterns because we were doing night shifts and frequent calls. I developed ulcerated and severe sores in my mouth. I was unable to smile at the end of the day because my mouth was so swollen and painful. On top of the pain, I was not able to eat. Everything, even water, burned my mouth. My tongue was raw. My joints hurt. I had strange itchy rashes on my legs, arms, and back. I lost weight rapidly, a total of eighteen pounds.

As if I needed more stress, at this same time, we had a huge flood, and we had the house repaired with big commercial fans and replacement of Sheetrock. The contractors discovered black mold in the bathroom wall, which was also torn out and remediated. Though now, I know this was not properly done.

> **Fast Fact**
>
> For some susceptible individuals, mycotoxin exposure is life threatening. For others, it can be a noxious stimuli for the immune system.[4]

For my erosive lichen planus, the specialists informed me there was no cure. I was offered steroids and a new biologic infusion that was so expensive that my PCP suggested we take out a second mortgage to cover the cost.

The cost was one consideration, but this time of year was the height of cold and flu season, and I was working at the Children's Hospital. One of the risks of this medication is progressive multifocal leukoencephalopathy (PML), most often a fatal attack on the brain secondary to a common virus. That didn't sound appealing to me.

I did the only thing I knew to do, go back to the basics. With supported gut health, I did the best I could with immune modulation. (I studied the disease process and which immune pathway was most involved.) I replaced nutrients and went heavy on the antioxidants. (Now I know why I did so well with glutathione supplementation. It has to do with my genetics. I will explain this in detail later.) I also did the best I could at removing and reducing my exposure to environmental toxicities and made my mental and spiritual well-being a priority.

And now in 2019, I can happily say I have been in full remission for ten years. I am not taking any routine prescription medications. I have had three small flares in the last nine years. I made it through business start-ups and job changes. I even made it through a year of hell. I discovered

---

[4] Winnie-Pui-Pui Liew and Sabran Mohd-Redzwan, "Mycotoxin: Its Impact on Gut Health and Microbiota," *Front Cell Infect Microbiol* 8(2018): 60, doi: 10.3389/fcimb.2018.00060 PMID: 29535978.

infidelity and endured the resulting divorce without a major setback. So there it is, my journey. I am glad you hung in there with me.

As you know, I did many things to get well, some not found in science and others strongly supported in prominent scientific literature. I do not know if there is one particular thing I did that was really the big turnkey; however, I will say all of it cumulatively served a purpose. I understand that everyone's body is different. We are complex unique creatures who thus require a unique approach to our health challenges.

To translate my life lessons into advice for you, the first, and in my opinion, the most important is diet, as you heard above. If I had to pick a second life-changing treatment, I would emphatically say deep breathing, quiet time, and honoring the body's needs. From a biochemical standpoint, the improvements in my internal health resulted from bowel health improvements, genetic support for biotransformation (detoxification), and restoration of immune balance.

In the following chapters, I will dive into the science behind such transformative treatments and give tools for clinical implementation. With clear approaches, you can tailor your treatments to the individual and watch as the systems work together to achieve homeostasis with proper support.

REFERENCES

1. J. Y. Lee, M. E. C. Abundo, C. W. Lee, "Herbal Medicines with Antiviral Activity Against the Influenza Virus, a Systematic Review," *Am J Chin Med* 46(8)(2018): 1663–1700.
2. Jiang-Hua Li, Zhi-Hui Wang, Xiao-Juan Zhu, Zhao-Hui Deng, Can-Xin Cai, Li-Qiang Qiu, Wei Chen, and Ya-Jun Lin, "Health Effects from Swimming Training in Chlorinated Pools and the Corresponding Metabolic Stress Pathways," *PLoS* 10(3)(March 5, 2015).

CHAPTER ONE

WHAT IS FUNCTIONAL MEDICINE? AND WHY?

I present this book to an intended audience of healers: physicians, physician assistants, nurse practitioners, nurses, dieticians, and health coaches, to name a few.

The idea of optimal function and patient improvement is really not farfetched. Why are we settling for mediocre practices and results? Most of us went into practice to help people. And yes, medicine has become a bit of a hassle from all the demands—electronic health records (EHR), prior authorization requests, and patient expectations that do not fit within insurance-driven reality.

But if you could see twenty to thirty people daily, as we do in a typical family outpatient clinic, and of those twenty to thirty, at least 50 to 70 percent were satisfied and grateful for you and your staff, would you not feel fulfilled at the end of the day? Achieving this rate of satisfaction is how we can overcome or survive physician burnout. So let me show you how you can practice medicine within its current outlines and have a true patient outcome improvement with a satisfaction rate greater than 60 percent.

One practical advantage for your practice is that healthier, happier patients are a constant source of referrals as they share their positive experiences. Patients do not want to sit in a waiting room for hours before they get to see a doctor for five minutes, and most often they wait to see a clinician who never once touches them, much less listens to their full range of concerns. I believe that we can change the face of medicine. Read with me so you can do what you love, heal people.

Before we get to the meat of this how-to book, I need to lay the foundation. First, what is functional medicine? I feel it necessary to spend some time on this subject because there is much confusion in the medical community between functional medicine and integrative medicine.

As per the Institute for Functional Medicine, the leader in clinician training, for this new approach to chronic disease, functional medicine is defined as a personalized, systems-oriented model that empowers patients and practitioners to achieve the highest expression of health by working in collaboration to address the underlying causes of disease.

As I journeyed through the world of alternative medicine and then osteopathic medicine and functional medicine, I heard it all. Functional medicine was, for me, the best means by which I could merge those two worlds of training. In all realms of life, we often see a "left or a right" following, as most people are uncomfortable with the gray area. I found this to be the case in both courses of medical training.

Too often I interacted with physicians and healers who were convinced their ways were the only truth. For example, many naturopaths believe prescription drugs are harmful, and many of my medical colleagues believe herbals to be anecdotal. And the others are "bad, inaccurate, or scary." And I have even heard declarations of a healing method being "evil."

It seems in most careers, especially medicine, we tend to implement what we are told, taught, and especially what we experience. There are many modalities of healing worldwide, and I appreciate and respect what may be your truth, even though what may work for you may not be the path for my patient or me. It is impossible for one person to master all methods of healing. If you cannot offer your patients what they need, the least you can do is respectfully support them on their journey.

Functional medicine was a way I could utilize principles from my alternative health training and apply the science and research of my medical training. I am honored to have been among the first eighty-eight certified functional medicine practitioners in the world. In 2001, we were the first graduating class of the Institute for Functional Medicine.

Functional medicine is an amazing approach to chronic disease and disease prevention based on biochemistry, physiology, and genetics, an area of medicine growing at an exponential rate with an increase of more than 50 percent in online searches over the last five years. The Institute for Functional Medicine had 1.6 million patient-initiated searches for functional medicine practitioners in 2018.[5]

Cleveland Clinic Center for Functional Medicine is setting a high standard for demonstrating that individualized, root-cause medicine can be cost effective for both patient and insurer. During my time as a clinician and leader with this group, I came to appreciate the challenge faced as a new systems-based model for chronic disease in replacing the acute-care model. This change is inevitable, especially if we expect to stop the health-care deficit.

Dr. Mark Hyman and Dr. Patrick Hanaway have taken the lead in making this vision a reality. Cleveland Clinic is the pioneering institution but soon won't be the only functional medicine center in the world. Despite the rapid influx of practitioners into this new field

---

[5] "The Institute for Functional Medicine Surpasses 1,000 IFM Certified Practitioners in Functional Medicine Globally," https://www.ifm.org/news-insights/ifm-surpasses-1000-certified-practitioners

of medicine, there are still not enough physicians in primary care and even less with functional medicine training for this worldwide demand.[6]

There are likely several reasons for this shortage. In my opinion, the primary is what I call the "payment-to-heart deficiency." If you are employed in an insurance-based practice and are lucky to be allowed the time it takes to practice functional medicine, you will not be properly reimbursed for the time needed to interview, formulate a plan, and refine treatment for your patient—the work of the heart. Often this lack of compensation leads clinicians to leave the insured medical practice to open a cash-based practice.

The problem I found was that the vast majority of patients cannot afford to see a health-care provider without insurance help. However, the education to become a physician is not cheap. I was $200,000 in debt for medical school and residency. As much as many clinicians would love to give away or barter for services, we have debts to pay. Many of us have a desire to help patients but lack the time to practice functional medicine within a system that is driven solely by revenue.

Recently published in the *Journal of American Medicine* (JAMA) was data demonstrating excellent patient outcomes with this model for chronic disease.[7] Proving to be great for patient health outcomes is great, but until insurance accepts and covers a functional medicine health-care model, I would like to offer a solution.

As an alternative to the cash-based practice of primary care, I propose a blended functional primary-care approach for insurance-based

---

[6] After you experience successes that fill your heart with joy and revitalize your love for medicine, you may decide to pursue a complete certification in functional medicine. Fellowship options or certifications can be found through the Institute for Functional Medicine (www.ifm.org).

[7] Michelle Beidelschies, PhD[1], Marilyn Alejandro-Rodriguez, BSAS[1], Xinge Ji, MS[2], et al., "Association of the Functional Medicine Model of Care with Patient-Reported Health-Related Quality-of-Life Outcomes," *JAMA* 2(10)(October 25, 2019), doi:e1914017. oi:10.1001.

practitioners. This model can benefit any provider who wants to offer more fulfilling patient-practitioner interaction on a daily basis. Regardless of your field of specialty, I hope the information in this book will help transform your practice into a rewarding experience for all involved.

HIS-TORY, HER-STORY, HISTORY

I spent more than five years in an outpatient family practice as an employee of a large hospital, where I learned how to incorporate my family and functional medicine training to offer my patients more options. There are several ways to help a patient, and the first suggestion on my list is basic: listen to the patient's story.

The clues are in the history, as we are taught in medical school. Listening and taking a good history is important to help direct the plan and differential. Listening starts the healing process, builds trust, and opens the door for more learning. If you are going to incorporate functional medicine into the interaction, this process is essential to the visit. However, because time is limited, both parties must be aware of this principle: the history must be conveyed concisely within the given amount of time.

Functional medicine requires more thought and thus more time. When the schedule does not budge, as patients, we must be concise in our delivery. As physicians, we must be astute to the patient's presentation and key points. Therefore, I suggest setting clear expectations at the beginning, starting with your front office staff and scheduling.

> **Tip**
>
> In setting expectations, remember that a true return to homeostasis is not going to happen overnight. It took the body many years to arrive at its current state, and treating the root cause takes effort and time. Be patient.

ORGANIZING

Second, functional medicine has a few fundamental tools that can help change your assessment of the patient's complaint or concern. The first of these tools is the matrix. The functional medicine matrix is a system-based wheel within which you can organize the patient's symptoms and signs, either mentally (for lack of time) or physically (EHR, either written or scanned).

The wheel allows you to see what system(s) most in need of attention are. System categories include defense and repair, assimilation, structural, communication, transport, biotransformation, and elimination and energy. (I reference the Institute for Functional Medicine training tools only including the matrix wheel.)

Examples of Complaints, Symptoms, or Signs in Each Matrix Category

Symptoms and signs may appear in multiple categories.

Assimilation: digestion, absorption, microbiome, respiration

Defense/Repair: immune system, inflammation, infection

Structural: musculoskeletal system, cellular membrane

Communication: neuroendocrine and immune systems

Transport: cardiovascular and lymphatic systems

Biotransformation: detoxification, toxicity

Energy: mitochondrial dysfunction, energy regulation

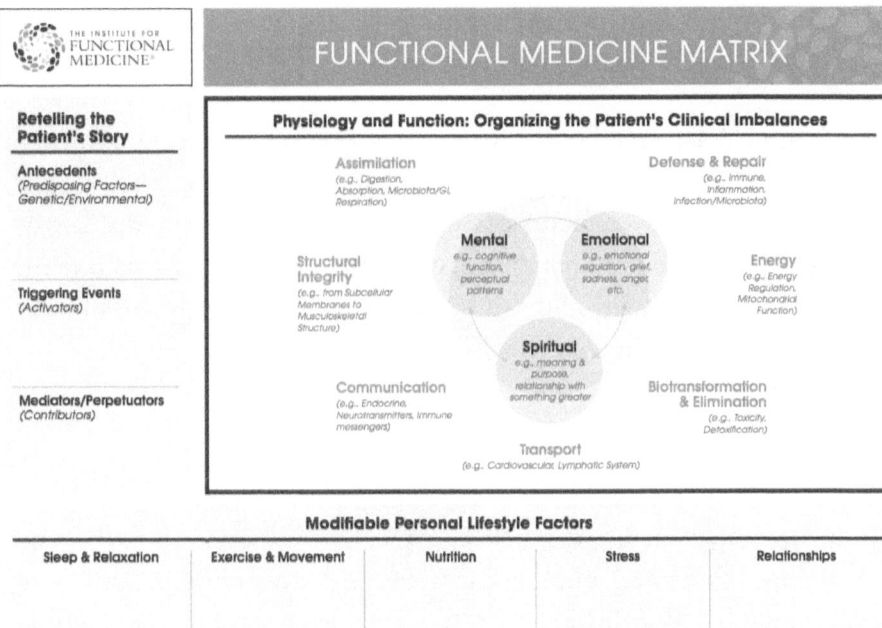

Matrix

A medical symptoms questionnaire (MSQ) is a compilation of symptoms the patient has experienced over a specified amount of time. Sometimes it is best to see how they have been over the last four to eight weeks instead of the last forty-eight hours or a lifetime. The questionnaire should be relative to the patient's presentation. (See appendix A for an example.)

It is helpful in implementation to establish the timeline. On paper or using a computer, have the patient complete a mental, physical, and spiritual health chronology from birth to the present. Don't overlook this simple tool. Hans Hoffman said, "The ability to simplify means to eliminate the unnecessary so that the necessary may speak."

The third and final basic, functional medicine application is the consistent appreciation of the patient's triggers, mediators, and antecedents. Triggers are actions, habits, and anything that could potentially elicit a change in homeostasis. Mediators are stimulants to the system, things that keep a response going.

Being in an abusive relationship or an ongoing exposure to environmental toxins and *even* constant inflammatory cytokine activity are all common examples of mediators. An antecedent is essentially family history. Genetics fall in this category. Document these points. Have the patient help you. By this, I mean I recommend you include this into the electronic medical records (EMR) intake process.

WHERE DOES THE TIME GO?

In a functional medicine practice, typically the physician will spend an average of one and a half hours with the patient at their initial visit exclusively to collect information and order appropriate tests as well as gather a comprehensive history from birth to the present. Well, isn't that nice, you say?

In standard primary care practice, we are lucky to get fifteen minutes with each patient. I, as do all physicians, understand the importance of the patient's story, but as I have said, in the current model, time limits us. So how do we solve this?

Fast Fact

7.6 minutes with a patient is the average reported initial primary care visit, and patients regularly announce the time they were speaking was less than five minutes.

My solution for the history-taking portion of a functional medicine primary care initial visit includes alternative means of obtaining information and highlighted application of knowledge to optimize

---

[8] A. D. Racine, "Providers and patients face-to-face: what is the time?" *Isr J Health Policy Res* 6, 54 (2017), doi:10.1186/s13584-017-0180-1.

health outcomes. I propose the initial visit still include a questionnaire and a chronological timeline of the patient's physical, emotional, and spiritual health from birth to current time, which should be specific to their chief complaint.

Patients can help the provider quickly analyze their history if it is concise, available before the appointment, and easy to read in chronological order. This allows the provider the ability to quickly assess the information without interruption before entering the room. Furthermore, a valuable physical exam can then be general or tailored to the complaint system(s).

In the office with the patient, ask a few point questions relative to the questionnaire and personal history derived from your quick review of their timeline. For example, if they are there for IBS symptoms, review your IBS questionnaire and their timeline and then gather more specific information from the area on timeline that you notice is a "high point area."

A high point area is an area on the chronological timeline that has a lot of activity, trauma, stress, illness, and so on, specifically an area you note where their health changed "took a turn for the worse." There's no need to discuss or engage in conversation around all the little details following or proceeding this hot spot (high point area).

Appreciate and read them, but do not focus on this. You can easily get wrapped up in the less pertinent information. You can always reflect. For example, if they are not getting better with your ongoing recommendations, bring them in for a visit, review the history again, and pay attention to the timeline. Stepping back, look for other triggers or mediators.

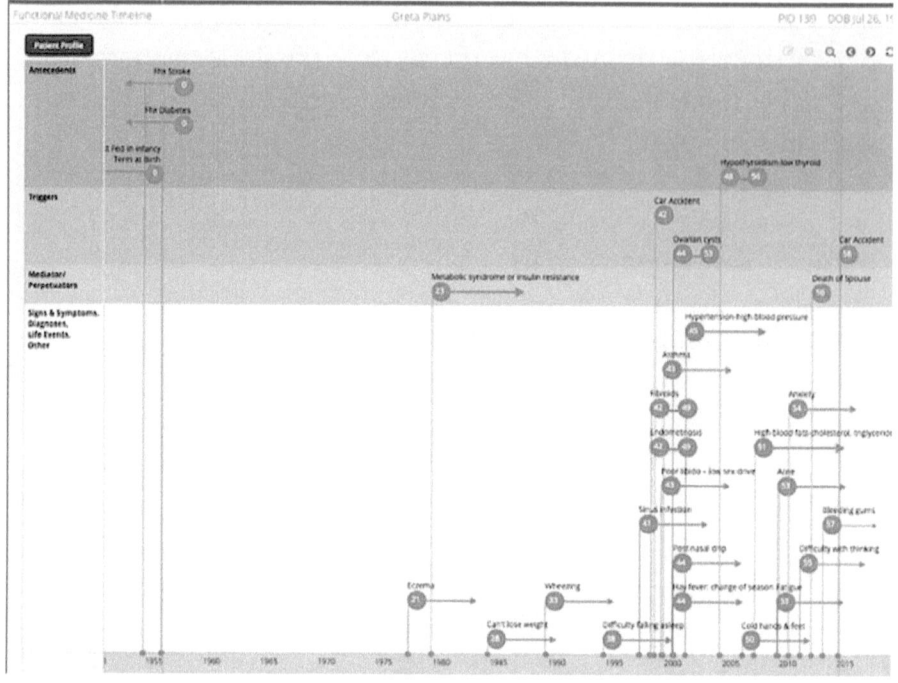

Timeline

What if they are there for a straightforward complaint, let's say an urinary tract infection (UTI), upper respiratory infection (URI), or back strain? When a patient presents with a common primary care complaint, just think about optimization of bodily function.

As a good example, a UTI, treat it and support the system. I recommend the patient limit sugar and baths for a week and increase water intake. Whole, fresh cranberries (or in pill form) can be added to the diet but only for short bursts.

In my experience, I saw many patients who were consuming too many capsules for too long, and this can change pH of urine and cause spasms, mimicking UTI symptoms. I use probiotics, especially increasing a patient's dietary intake. Research literature is mixed on this recommendation, but I find it helpful. If they have chronic UTIs, start asking why? Hormones or lack thereof? Change in pH? Diet? High blood glucose?

> **Fast Fact**
>
> For UTIs, a cranberry cocktail is not helpful! Cranberry concentrate, the kind that makes you pucker, has been proven to help reduce the risk of UTIs, not treat an ongoing infection, because the proanthocyanins interfere with the bacteria's ability to adhere to the bladder wall (American Journal of Obstetrics and Gynecology 2015).

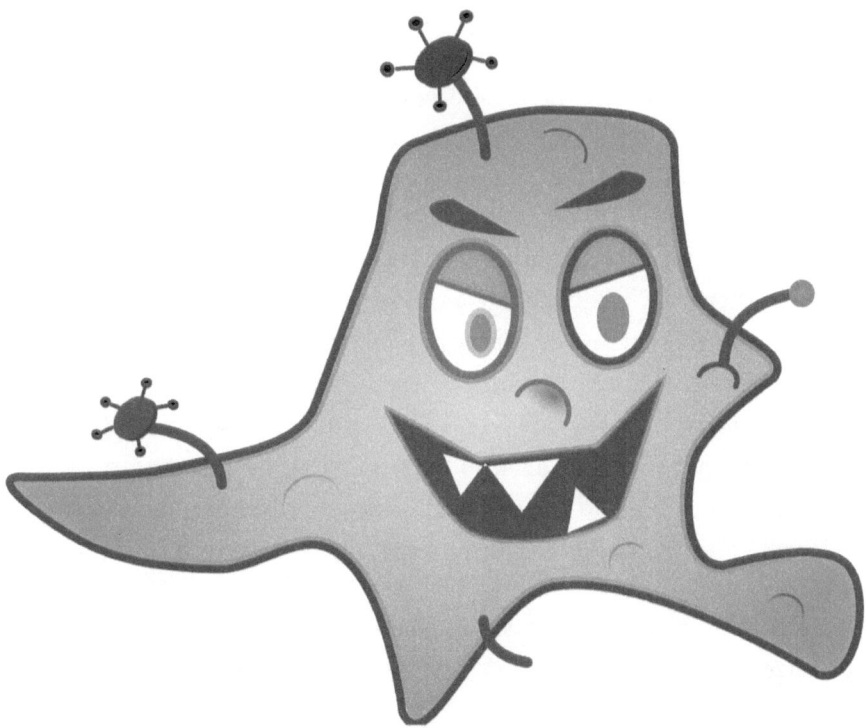

Another example of a straightforward visit is upper respiratory infections, sore throats, and viral illnesses. Simply said, support the system. Rest, water, veggie juices, herbal teas, and time in the sauna is part of my repertoire. Patients do not have to leave with a prescription of antibiotics if you have something else to offer and you reassure them it is a virus. We are in an era of multiple drug resistance infections because of overprescribing and wrongful treatment of viral illnesses with antibiotics. Antibiotics are warranted when necessary, especially when patients do not improve with conservative treatments, for instance, persistent fever and/or worsening of symptoms.

(Pic from applegate.com)

Another example, which is a little less simplistic but a common complaint, is fatigue. My first recommendation for these patients is to optimize thyroid function. If they are complaining of fatigue and thyroid-stimulating hormone (TSH) is normal, try checking the rest of the biochemical/pathophysiological markers that we have available to us: free T3, free T4, the antibodies thyroglobulin and microsomal, and so on. This will give you a better appreciation of the thyroid functionality, not just how the pituitary is stimulating the thyroid.

Recall that TSH is a stimulating hormone reacting in response to a stimulus (negative feedback). Make sure when you get your patient's results back, they are all in the middle to normal range and that it is consistent with the TSH results. If there is a mismatch, for instance, if there is a low free T4, low free T3, elevated reverse T3, and TSH is normal, the negative feedback loop is going to be influenced by that elevated reverse T3, and the physical symptoms and presentation of the patient is more of fatigue because of the low free thyroid hormones.[9]

There is more to come on this topic later. Nevertheless, the point is to optimize function.

---

[9] Yasaman Pirahanchi and Ishwarlal Jialal, "Physiology, Thyroid Stimulating Hormone (TSH)," https://www.ncbi.nlm.nih.gov/books/NBK499850

LET'S PUT IT TOGETHER!

First and foremost, optimization of function should be addressed with lifestyle and diet. As far as lifestyle is concerned, the patient must be aware of the importance of nurturing their mental well-being with community support or respecting their need for quiet time by learning to say no.

Equally important is diet. Feeding their bodies with a balanced, clean diet and staying hydrated is an area we as practitioners can educate frequently. Never forget to ensure healthy sleep habits and how all this affects their health. Then they will understand the value of this key element.

Simply assure these points are addressed first, and most of all your patients will have some improvement. This discussion at the first encounter also sets the stage for the patient expectation. I cannot adequately express the value of this conversation. Establishing a relationship requires a foundation of expectations.

This does not mean there is no room for growth and flexibility, but they won't be offended if they show up for a viral illness complaint and you recommend rest, a hot bath, or sauna time and ginger tea, assuring you will avoid the "no antibiotics" question. Most always, I find with the education of these lifestyle habits, your patients will need less of the expensive testing and medications.

CASE EXAMPLE

A simple case study is the best way to demonstrate what one might expect at a visit. This case presentation is a patient who presents with a chief complaint of migraines, a common complaint for primary care, and the first-line medications are expensive and not curative.[10]

Mrs. White presents as a thirty-five-year-old female with a twenty-year history of migraines. Mrs. White hoped to see Dr. FunctionalGP because she had heard many people in town speaking about regained health. Mrs. White called into the office and was pleasantly greeted by the staff, who as part of the scheduling process requested Mrs. White either log into the practice's secure website and fill out her information, including a timeline, or come early to do it in the office.

If her chief complaint required a more comprehensive evaluation, the scheduling staff added a kind comment, such as "the better you fill the timeline with important mental, physical, and spiritual stressors from birth to now, the better our clinicians will be able to help you." This set the pretense. They also advised the patient it may be necessary to accomplish her goal in stages, which may require a few visits. Again, expectations—established up front—is key!

You may feel it helpful, if Mrs. White is challenged by technology, that she bring her timeline by the office before her visit at least one or two days prior. Some patients will bring it to their visit, but this may mean the clinician has to spend precious time reading it before they are able to commence with the face-to-face visit.

I would review her timeline, taking time to note important triggers or mediators if I have it ahead of time. Quickly I reviewed it, mentally noting systems that are of heavy concern. However, in this example, with Mrs. White, I received her information before the visit, so I mentally noted systems of heavy concern on the matrix: energy (migraines, insomnia), assimilation (IBS), and biotransformation (migraines).

---

[10] W. J. Becker, "The Diagnosis and Management of Chronic Migraine in Primary Care," *Headache* 57(9)(2017): 1471–1481.

This took me about two minutes. This could be done outside her door if in a rush. Once reviewed, I entered her room, and after a bit of introduction and conversation, I began my physical exam. All the while, I asked pertinent questions regarding her timeline. If I were lucky, I would have a scribe enter these pertinent points. If not, at the end of my physical exam, I would enter this information into my EHR. Interestingly, for Mrs. White, current age of thirty-five, I noted a drastic change in her health around the age of ten. So I will start here.

The conversation would sound something like this.

Doctor: Mrs. White, I noticed at the age of ten you started having headaches regularly, and at that time, you also started having stomach pains, cramping, and constipation. What was happening in your life at this time?

Mrs. White: We moved to the country, and life was good on a farm. We raised our own animals.

Doctor: Mrs. White, did your diet change drastically? Was there ever a period of your life when you did not have migraines or they improved?

With this inquisition, Mrs. White revealed a new exposure to whole milk.

Mrs. White: We made our own butter and so on.

She also disclosed multiple tick bites. Mrs. White admitted her sleep changed around this time as well. She said she "could not sleep and woke extremely early."

WORKUP

Assimilation and energy (categories of the matrix above) were her primary focus points (ongoing IBS and fatigue). Therefore, my recommendation would be to work on the assimilation and digestion and assess for food allergies and sensitivities. And for the energy section, I would check thyroid function (as hypothyroidism can cause constipation and headaches) and nutrient levels associated with constipation and headaches (e.g., magnesium, zinc, calcium and Omega-3 index). My two- to four-minute exam revealed a scalloped, large, red tongue, leukonychia on most fingernails (thus the reason for zinc and calcium levels), and rough, dry skin (omega-3s and vitamin A).

Next, the relative labs were ordered via EHR, and the visit was over. I explained to Mrs. White that we would start here and review the results at the next visit. In the meantime, I recommended two very important lifestyle modifications in addition to her lab draw, which I printed on her plan.

PLAN #1

I asked that she undergo a dietary change, a basic reset. By this, I recommended she increase her dark green intake, reduce her sugar and caffeine consumption, and ensure eight to ten glasses of water per day. I suggest you meet your patient where they are. For example, if they are vegans and eat clean, then no change is needed until test results are back, and if they eat nothing but Starbucks and fast food, then add a green vegetable with two meals per day and reduce the coffee intake to one cup per day.

Her test results would include Immunoglobulin G (IgG) food testing, which allowed me to tailor her eating plan accordingly.

PLAN #2

I asked that she start a mindfulness practice each morning. (In this case, mindfulness consisted of fifteen minutes of breathing-focused guided meditation.) And since she was going to high-impact aerobics five times per week, I asked her to reduce that to two times per week. For the other three days, she would do meditative walking for twenty to forty minutes with some stretching.

Her reaction to this request was all too familiar. "Why? I thought exercise was good for me!"

I responded with a quick explanation about the need to decrease inflammation and restore mitochondrial function.

That is it! You are done!

Your seven- to fifteen-minute visit was a success for your patient and you. You may be the first healer to have inquired about her life story, and you most likely will be the only one to look for a root cause to her migraines. This initial visit took approximately fifteen minutes—longer if you wish and are able to review the timeline in detail—but for the sake of limited office visits as outlined by insurance demands, I have demonstrated how a physician can still incorporate functional medicine into the daily new patient encounters.

FOLLOW-UP VISIT

With the initial visit aside, my follow-up encounter with Mrs. White ensued four weeks later. Her IgG food sensitivity panel revealed abnormal results to dairy and corn. She reported her bowels had improved with the water increase and the dark green intake but were still not regular. We discussed the relativeness of IgG versus Immunoglobulin E (IgE) food reactions. IgG is an immune reaction, "delayed type four response." It does not mean she is allergic.[11]

---

[11] H. Tlaskalová-Hogenová, L. Tucková, R. Stepánková, T. Hudcovic, L. Palová-Jelínková, and N. Y. Ann, "Involvement of innate immunity in the development of inflammatory and autoimmune diseases," Acad Sci 1051(2005): 787–798, PMID: 16127016, DOI: 10.1196/annals.1361.122.

Often I explain with verbiage similar to this: "For you, Mrs. White, these foods are merely adding to the inflammatory response every time you ingest dairy and corn." Many proteins cause antibody responses in the human body, and a general "IgG cow's milk" is not specific to casein or caesomorphin.

So in lieu of this knowledge, for all patients whom test similarly, I simply recommend avoidance of all dairy for a period of time. I start with a specified eight to twelve weeks. Then with the help of a dietician, reintroduce and adjust according to clinical response.

Mrs. White was referred to a dietician at this point in the treatment plan. (This is not always necessary, and often patients cannot afford this added service. Fortunately insurance covers it, particularly if you can identify vitamin deficiencies, diabetes, and so forth.) All other labs were reviewed, and a follow-up was scheduled for eight weeks.

This was a full fifteen- to twenty-minute follow-up with a limited physical exam. I recommend having the dietician or your staff check in on your patient one or two times before the next follow-up, if possible. It could even be a simple email or text, again a short and sweet interaction.

For Mrs. White, a second follow-up was scheduled for me to assess her clinical response. Most presentations get better with the basics. If your patient is not improving and you have reached your training maximum for functional medicine, then refer to a functional medicine practitioner who can dive further into other etiologies. If you refer, your patient will not leave you.

As a matter of fact, most of the time, I find the practitioner to whom you refer your patient will become part of your patient's care team. I believe this happens because you have been attentive and caring, which ultimately ensures a healthy relationship with the patient. As a result, they will not only thank you for the referral, but feel secure in the knowledge they have a team.

I have been practicing functional/integrative medicine for more than nineteen years, and I can say I am constantly humbled and constantly learning. I tell my patients they are at the mercy of my learning curve. I will do my best, and I know when I need to ask for expert opinion. I know when I need to refer.

Now that the foundation for an office visit has been laid, I want to offer some of what I have learned, areas in primary care I feel we can impact patient outcomes with some basic functional medicine application.

CHAPTER TWO

LIFESTYLE MODIFICATION: DIET, EXERCISE, AND SAUNA

LIFESTYLE MODIFICATIONS

Lifestyle modification is the simplest yet most accessible clinical application for significant health improvement. This includes proper rest, quiet time, and deep breathing. (I even recommend this be separate from prayer because often in prayer, we are praying for someone whom we are worried about.) This is important but not considered "deep breathing or meditation time" (as worry increases sympathetic fight-or-flight cascades.)

> **Fast Fact**
>
> More than 80 percent of chronic conditions could be avoided through the adoption of healthy lifestyle recommendations.[12]

---

[12] I. Jialal and U. Rajamani. "Endotoxemia of metabolic syndrome: a pivotal mediator of meta-inflammation," *Metab Syndr Relat Disord* 12(9)(2014): 454–456, DOI: 10.1089.

SLEEP AND REST

As we all know—and it should go without saying—sleep is vital to excellent health. If we can get our patients to have deep restorative sleep nightly, we can assure healing and restoration. Melatonin has mixed reviews in the scientific literature, and the meta-analysis journal published in 2014 suggests, based on multiple well-performed studies, though most small in size, melatonin is a category B recommendation for insomnia and jet lag, but category C for shift work sleep disorders.[1]

I do advise my patients that the research is limited for several reasons, but one of the most significant flaws, in my opinion, is the melatonin used is not identified as immediate release versus slow release. Melatonin is not particularly effective producing quick-onset sleep. It is best used to increase deep-restorative sleep. And melatonin has a short half-life in the immediate form, so I find slow-release melatonin to be more effective. Avoidance of blue light before bed and assuring daily sunlight exposure is also an effective means of increasing one's own melatonin production.

Pyridoxal phosphate, P-5-P, the active form of B6, and magnesium are also very important nutrients in the biochemical conversion from tryptophan to melatonin.

Fast Fact

Melatonin is also helpful when trying to wean off acid blockers and proton pump inhibitors.[13]

Sleep is important! But rest is just as important. Deep breathing, meditation, or quiet time throughout the day is an extremely effective

---

[13] J. Tan, Y. Wang, Y. Xia, N. Zhang, X. Sun, T. Yu, and Lin, "Melatonin protects the esophageal epithelial barrier by suppressing the transcription, expression and activity of myosin light chain kinase through ERK1/2 signal transduction," *Cell Physiol Biochem* 34(6)(2014): 2117–2127, DOI: 10.1159/000369656.

means of dampening the sympathetic (fight-or-flight) response in the body. Fifteen to twenty minutes in the afternoon is ideal. For most, between 1:00 and 3:00 p.m. can improve immune regulation, sleep, and mood. And it is free!

I recommend you suggest your patient go to a quiet room at work and put their head down, with no TV, phone, music, computer, or friends ... nothing. Just relaxing, deep breathing. (They can have calm, no-word music as a timer, assuring they do not fall and stay asleep.) It will be a challenge, especially at first, for many.

Let the mind wander and race. Just return to the breath and keep the body relaxed. I started doing this in residency, for instance, in my car in the parking garage. I continued in private practice with a floor mat rolled out on the floor and a sticky note on the door. And I still do this as a hospitalist, usually in my car. (I must share my experience. A note worded "napping" was not a deterrent to those "needing me," but a note on the door, "meditating and praying," proved most effective in preventing a knock.)

Additionally I recommend ten to fifteen minutes of meditation/mindfulness in the morning. I trained myself to relax using a free guided mindfulness app. It took about a year, and now I do not need any guidance. I prefer to sit on my couch and do this, but life is life. Sometimes I do it before I get out of my car and head into work. I make it a daily priority.

Science has proven regular meditation increases communication between hemispheres of the brain (makes us smarter) and improves immune regulation. It is also applicable for autoimmune disorders. See chapter 3 for details of improved immune regulation and a few more techniques and tools.

DIET

Let food be thy medicine! As it is and should be. Diet is one of the most important treatments I recommend for my patients, and this plan is most always tailored to the individual. There are many diets, for instance, food plans and trendy eating suggestions. What's my advice? Eat when you are hungry, avoid excess anything, do not eat refined sugar, avoid processed food, and listen to your body.

And when needed, seek the expert opinion of a registered dietician. As for an eating plan, there are several, and I would suggest we physicians (unless you have been trained as a dietitian) refer our patients for two primary reasons:

1. Because it is important.
2. Because of the limited time in an office visit, we really cannot do an excellent job formulating an eating plan for each of our patients.

I feel it is important to explain the difference, as I see it, between dietician and nutritionist. Then I would like to introduce the concept of functional nutritionist. Keep in mind that I am not an expert in this field. As a naturopath, I studied and had a special interest in nutrition, but I am neither certified nor licensed.

Registered dietitians (RD) have met the criteria set forth by the Commissions on Dietetics, and standard practice is based on the current government and medical food guidelines. A nutritionist does not require a minimum four-year degree and is not governed by continuing medical education. Functional registered dietitians and functional nutritionists have extra-functional medical nutrition training. Most RDs I know have at least master-level training (six years), and several have online practices.

I recommend you introduce yourself to a RD or two and refer your patients to them often. However, the Mediterranean diet and the plant-based eating plans[14] are a good place to start most people.[15] Just getting rid of diet beverages and refined sugar as well as limiting caffeine and alcohol to occasional use will be dramatic dietary changes that will result in huge improvements.

TIP

A diet high in prebiotic foods and probiotics for most is a must. From an article in Healthline,

> Evidence shows that many chronic metabolic diseases do arise in the gut. Your gut bacteria and the integrity of your gut lining strongly affect your health. According to numerous studies, undesirable bacterial products called endotoxins can sometimes leak through your gut lining and enter your bloodstream. Your immune system then recognizes these foreign molecules and attacks them—resulting in chronic inflammation. Some hypothesize that this diet-induced inflammation may trigger insulin and leptin resistance—driving factors for type 2 diabetes and obesity, respectively. It's also believed to cause fatty liver disease. At the very least, inflammation has been strongly linked to many of the world's most serious conditions. [9,10,11,12,13]

---

[14] You can obtain information for the Mediterranean and plant-based eating plans at https://www.hsph.harvard.edu/nutritionsource/healthy-weight/diet-reviews/mediterranean-diet.

[15] Philip J. Tuso, MD, "Nutritional Update for Physicians: Plant-Based Diets," Perm J 17(2)(2013): 61–66, PMCID: PMC3662288, PMID: 23704846, DOI: 10.7812/TPP/12-085.

MOVEMENT

Similar to diet recommendations, treatment plans for exercise are individual, and it is okay to start with meditative, mindful walking. That is easy enough.

Take a relaxing, calm walk with a focus on your breath. I ask my patients to increase every week or two the time it takes them to complete the distance they walked the week before or increase the distance all together.

Core strength is also very important, as it improves posture and thus eases back strain. Plank holds are easy enough to start. Start slow and low. Seek the advice of a professional, if needed. Adapt any exercise to fit the person and their capabilities.

Silver Sneakers for my more mature patients is a prescription given regularly. Balance is key to fall prevention. Balance poses are easy enough to recommend, even for the weak and wobbly. They can use the aid of the wall and/or a chair/sofa. Stretching is also important, especially as we age or if we are very active. Pick a few favorites, add them to the ones above, hand out a piece of paper to your patients, and circle their homework.

For aerobic exercise, advance as tolerated. Offer incentives. Earn a T-shirt if your personal trainer signs proof of activity or your Zumba instructor writes that you attended x number classes. Make it fun! Heck, there are even apps for Zombie runs and games you can play on your walk. Just get your patients moving!

As for the philosophy, "exercise is the answer to every ailment," I disagree. This may seem redundant, but because it is so important and in such opposition to our training, it begs repetition. My severely fatigued and mitochondrial debilitated patients get worse with increased activity.

So with this small population, I start with nutrient replacement and deep breathing. Then I cautiously add in exercise for this patient population. Personally, I went from a type-A athlete, always active, to exhausted and barely able to dress myself. And had you told me, "Just exercise and you'll feel better," I would have thrown some choice words your direction ... silently.

Nonetheless, for my health, it would have been the worst thing I could do at that time. May I remind you that I was nutrient deplete, and any exercise meant more oxidative stress in the form of reactive oxidative species at a time when I did not have the capacity to recover from such a hit. I can attest this is true. I tried to exercise the pain and fatigue away. I was raised in the "no pain, no gain" era. Exercise only made me worse.

My well-meaning doctor's advice caused my muscle soreness—not to mention my exhaustion—to increase, and it lasted for days. Now I am very active. I exercise and walk daily. I love hiking, yoga, and gentle weight training.

So, clinicians, my advice is to be patient and adopt the same philosophy as I have shared with you. Each person is a unique individual, and their treatment should reflect this, An exercise prescription should be included. Meet them where they are.

For many of my patients, especially those unable to physically exercise, I often recommend the dry sauna as an alternate low-impact form of exercise. As you will see, sauna can be a multifaceted tool in your health plan.

SAUNA

For me, I feel sauna helped me in two ways:

1. I sweat. (I used to not be able to sweat. I just turned bright red.) And the more I sweat, the more I cleared toxins.

2. I increased the production of mitochondria, thus improving my energy levels.

Sauna, if the patient is medically capable to sit in a dry or infrared sauna, is highly recommended. My preference is a far infrared. The increase in temperature can improve their immune function. Sweating is detoxifying and helps with sore muscles and joints.

Scientists at the University of Eastern Finland are known for their research in sauna and health correlations. Information recently released from this group of respected scientists demonstrated the whys of sauna health benefits for lowering blood pressure and increasing vascular compliance.[16]

Sound familiar? This is what happens when a person performs a moderately intense workout! (Sauna is not a substitution for exercise, but this is why I use it for some patients who cannot exercise temporarily for whatever reason.)

The second finding was the decrease in pulse wave of 1.2 m/s, which over time has proven to decrease vessel stiffness. These findings were published in the *Journal of Human Hypertension*. The findings relating to the carotid-femoral pulse wave velocity measurements were published in the *European Journal of Preventive Cardiology*.

According to an article published in *JAMA* in 2015, sauna use of eleven to twenty minutes decreased sudden death from cardiac arrest in men by more than 52 percent compared to those who did not use saunas regularly. (This study defined regular use as three times per week.)[17]

---

[16] Joy Hussain and Marc Cohen, "Clinical Effects of Regular Dry Sauna Bathing: A Systematic Review," *Evid Based Complement Alternat Med* (2018): 1857413, doi.org/10.1155/2018/1857413.

[17] Tanjaniina Laukkanen, Hassan Khan, Francesco Zaccardi, and Jari A. Laukkanen, "Association Between Sauna Bathing and Fatal Cardiovascular and All-Cause Mortality Events," *JAMA Internal Medicine* (2015), DOI: 10.1001/jamainternmed.2014.8187.

The group that sat in a dry sauna for less than nineteen minutes only decreased their risk by 7 percent.

The relationship between regular sauna use and brain health has also made headlines in published research literature. More than two thousand men were followed over two decades, and even after several other health risk factors were accounted for, including age, exercise, and socioeconomic status, they reported a 66 percent reduction in dementia. Of course, the results can be attributed to all the physiologic cardiovascular benefits mentioned above, but they have also found an increase in brain-derived neurotrophic factor (BDNF), a stimulant known to increase neuronal growth and repair.[18]

As for my fibromyalgia and chronic fatigue patients, sauna is one of my number-one tools. These patients have a hard time being compliant to exercise. Any exercise seems to increase their fatigue and seriously compound their muscle pain.

Starting slowly, I recommend near infrared sauna (see below for differences between near and far infrared) as a means of simulating exercise. As their health improves, they naturally increase their exercise. It is a very effective tool. Core temperature increases and stimulates adenosine triphosphate (ATP) production in mitochondrial. The stimulation of ATP is elicited by the low wavelengths of near infrared absorbing into chromophores of cellular water and mitochondria. This stimulates cytochrome c oxidase (CCO) of the electron transport chain, thus increasing ATP. As a result, slowly their energy increases, as does their ability to heal and repair through improved immune function and biotransformation.[19]

---

[18] Tanjaniina Laukkanen, Setor Kunutsor, Jussi Kauhanen, and Jari Antero Laukkanen, "Sauna bathing is inversely associated with dementia and Alzheimer's disease in middle-aged Finnish men," *Age and Ageing* 46 (2)(2017): 245–249, doi.org/10.1093/ageing/afw212

[19] K. Matsushita, A. Masuda, and C. Tei, "Efficacy of Infrared Sauna Therapy for Fibromyalgia," *Internal Medicine* 47(16)(2008): 1473–1476.

> **Fast Fact**
>
> Many patients tend to be nutrient deplete, especially in minerals like magnesium. A pinch of mineral salt and magnesium replacement before the sauna time or right after is helpful, especially if they demonstrate magnesium deficiency signs.

Most of the literature references far infrared sauna, heat at approximately 100 degrees Fahrenheit. The health benefits are astounding, but there is also near infrared sauna experiences with additional benefits. Near infrared penetrates your tissue more effectively for medical purposes than near infrared because wavelengths are under 900 nanometers (nm).[20],[21]

Dr. Alexander Wunsch nicely explains,

> Here you have only very low absorption by water molecules, and this is the reason why radiation has a very high transmittance. In other words, it penetrates

---

[20] Joseph Mercola, "How to Achieve Superior Detoxification and Health Benefits With Near-Infrared Light," Interview with Dr. Brian Richards, September 3, 2018. Shang-Ru Tsai, PhD, and Michael R Hamblin, PhD, "Biological effects and medical applications of infrared radiation," *J Photochem Photobiol B* 170(2017): 197–207, PMCID: PMC5505738, NIHMSID: NIHMS870595, PMID: 28441605, DOI: 10.1016/j.jphotobiol.2017.04.014.

[21] Fatma Vatansever and Michael R. Hamblin, "Far infrared radiation (FIR): its biological effects and medical applications," *Photonics Lasers Med* 4(2012): 255–266, DOI: 10.1515/plm-2012-0034, PMCID: PMC3699878, NIHMSID: NIHMS426504, PMID: 23833705.

very deeply into your tissue, so the energy distributes in a large tissue volume ... near-infrared A is not heating up the tissue so you will not feel directly any effect of heat. This significantly changes when we increase the wavelength, let's say, to 2,000 nm. Here we are in the infrared-B range and this already is felt as heat. And from 3,000 nm on to the longer wavelength, we have almost full absorption, mainly by the water molecule, and this is [felt as] heating.[22]

So I am not sure if it's the physiologic effects of the heat and sweating alone or if it is the fact that these people also were slowing down and relaxing for twenty minutes, but either way, sauna time proves to be time well spent.

Overall, lifestyle modification continues to be the first-line treatment for most disease prevention and treatment, and as you can see, modifying one's lifestyle must be tailored and can include many modalities.

RESOURCES FOR DIET, EXERCISE, AND SAUNA

1. Rebecca B Costello, et al., "The effectiveness of melatonin for promoting healthy sleep: a rapid evidence assessment of the literature," *Nutr J* 13(2014): 106., DOI: 10.1186/1475-2891-13-106, PMCID: PMC4273450, PMID: 25380732.
2. J. Tan, Y. Wang, Y. Xia, N. Zhang, X. Sun, T. Yu, and Lin, "Melatonin protects the esophageal epithelial barrier by suppressing the transcription, expression and activity of myosin light chain kinase through ERK1/2 signal transduction," *Cell Physiol Biochem* 34(6)(2014): 2117–2127, DOI: 10.1159/000369656.

---

[22] "How LED Lighting May Compromise Your Health," https://globalpossibilities.org/how-led-lighting-may-compromise-your-health-3.

3. I. Brzozowska, "Mechanisms of esophageal protection, gastroprotection and ulcer healing by melatonin. Implications for the therapeutic use of melatonin in gastroesophageal reflux disease (GERD) and peptic ulcer disease," Curr Pharm Des 20(30)(2014): 4807–4815.
4. Tanjaniina Laukkanen, Hassan Khan, Francesco Zaccardi, and Jari A. Laukkanen, "Association Between Sauna Bathing and Fatal Cardiovascular and All-Cause Mortality Events," *JAMA Internal Medicine* (2015), DOI: 10.1001/jamainternmed.2014.8187.
5. Tanjaniina Laukkanen, Setor Kunutsor, Jussi Kauhanen, and Jari Antero Laukkanen, "Sauna bathing is inversely associated with dementia and Alzheimer's disease in middle-aged Finnish men," *Age and Ageing* 46(2)(2017): 245–249.
6. Joy Hussain and Marc Cohen, "Clinical Effects of Regular Dry Sauna Bathing: A Systematic Review," *Evid Based Complement Alternat Med* (2018): 1857413.
7. A. D. Lopez and C. C. Murray, "The global burden of disease, 1990–2020," *Nat Med* 4(11)(1990): 1241–1243.
8. I. Jialal and U. Rajamani, "Endotoxemia of metabolic syndrome: a pivotal mediator of meta-inflammation," *Metab Syndr Relat Disord* 12(9)(2014): 454–456.
9. Pietro Vajro, et al., "Microbiota and gut liver axis: A Mini-Review on Their Influences on Obesity nd Obesity Related Liver Disease," *J Pediatr Gastroenterol Nutr* 56(5)(2013): 461–468.
You can obtain information for the Mediterranean and plant-based eating plans at https://www.hsph.harvard.edu/nutritionsource/healthy-weight/diet-reviews/mediterranean-diet and Perm J. 2013 Spring; 17(2): 61–66. DOI: 10.7812/TPP/12-085, PMCID: PMC3662288, PMID: 23704846.
Philip J. Tuso, MD, *Nutritional Update for Physicians: Plant-Based Diets.*

CHAPTER THREE

CFS: AKA SYSTEMIC EXERTION INTOLERANCE DISEASE (SEID) OR MYALGIC ENCEPHALOMYELITIS (ME)

Not being able to do more than one chore per day for fear it would result in twenty-four hours of bedrest was a reality for me at one time. Getting dressed and taking a shower was often too much for me. Now I exercise, work twelve hours, and come home, make dinner, and paint without exhaustion,

A common and daunting presenting complaint in a PCP's office is fatigue. If your patient has had significant complaints of fatigue for more than six months, the CDC diagnostic guideline (see the CDC questionnaire PDF in the resources) recommends you do a complete physical exam and thorough patient symptom review to assess for a diagnosis of chronic fatigue syndrome (CFS), myalgic encephlomylitis (ME), or systemic exertion intolerance disease (SEID).

ME is a multisystem-based chronic illness, which, for most, has a complex etiology. Not very well understood, the pathophysiology is relatively new in the literature, and several causes have been identified—infectious, genetic, and environmental—which individually and combined can contribute to a patient's presentation of CFS. The one agreed-upon pathogenesis is a trigger (most often an infection) of the immune B cell lineage, which alters the TH1/th2 response.[23] And long-term stimulation studies have shown the immune dysfunction affecting the brain and body of these patients. Unfortunately it is also very common for these same patients to present later with other syndromes, for instance, positional orthostatic tachycardia syndrome (POTS), fibromyalgia, and thyroid autoimmune disorders, to name a few.[24]

It is believed, once the trigger elicits an oxidative stress cascade, "The major immediate causes of the dysfunction are lack of essential substrates and partial blocking of the translocator protein sites in mitochondria."[25] Shy of diagnosing CFS and kindly sending them out the door with a "just exercise" prescription, we, as physicians, really don't have a lot to offer. CFS has neither definitive treatment nor cure as it stands. Supportive care and some off-label treatments are the current mainstream approach for patients who meet the criteria (also a bit controversial).

Immune-modulating medications like Inosine Pranobex (approved for use in several countries outside the US) and Rintatolimod are not available to those of us practicing in the United States yet. Rintatolimid has achieved statistically significant improvements in phase II and phase III double-blind, randomized, placebo-controlled clinical trials in the United States and Europe but will not see time on the shelf any time soon. Nonetheless, this is huge in the progress of CFS, not only because

---

[23] A. W. Taylor-Robinson and R. S. Phillips, "B cells are required for the switch from Th1- to Th2-regulated immune responses to Plasmodium chabaudi infection," *Infect Immun* 62(6)(1994): 2490–2498, PMID: 8188374, PMCID: PMC186536.

[24] Sarah J. Kizilbash, MD, Shelley P. Ahrens, RN, CNP, DNP, Barbara K. Bruce, PhD, Gisela Chelimsky, MD, et al., "Adolescent Fatigue, POTS, and Recovery: A Guide for Clinicians," *Curr Probl Pediatr Adolesc Health Care* 44(5)(2014): 108–133, PMID: 24819031, DOI: 10.1016/j.cppeds.2013.12.014.

[25] Boone et al., "Mitochondrial dysfunction and the pathophysiology of Myalgic Encephalomyelitis/Chronic Fatigue Syndrome (ME/CFS)," *Int J Clin Exp Med* 5(3) (2012): 208–20, PMID: 22837795, PMCID: PMC3403556.

there may be medicines to offer but also support for the diagnosis of this syndrome as an immune system dysregulation. Patients have gone for years feeling like "it was all in their head," even though I admit CFS is still veiled with a psychological undertone.

Personally, I can say it is so healing to receive validation and reassurance "it is not all in your head." Having the one person you sought to help you (your doctor) tell you it's all in your head and nothing is wrong simply because all your tests are normal is daunting and deflating.

After several encounters of this nature, the patient can most certainly add a component of hopelessness to their clinical presentation of fatigue and brain fog and, after an extended period, maybe even depression. It was difficult for me to hear "there is nothing wrong with you" time after time, without it affecting my psyche. Though fueled by my desire to be well and my determination to figure it out, I fought and used my frustration to regain my health.

Fast Fact

As early as 1969, research acknowledged Epstein–Barr virus (EBV) may not be the only trigger, and because the clinical acknowledgement lagged so poorly, the CDC launched a national education program in 2006.[26]

WHAT IS ONE TO DO WITH THE CFS DIAGNOSIS?

So now that we know CFS is a billable ICD-10, clinical diagnosis, what can we do for our patients? As I mentioned above, since CFS immune modulation with medication is not yet available to us in the United States, I propose we approach these patients with functional medicine.

---

[26] Elizabeth R. Unger, PhD, MD[1], Jin-Mann Sally Lin, PhD[1], Dana J. Brimmer, PhD, et al., "DC Grand Rounds: Chronic Fatigue Syndrome — Advancing Research and Clinical Education," *Weekly* 65(5051)(2016): 1434–1438.

I like to think of it in steps. The step at the base is the etiology/trigger: primary, secondary, and tertiary causes. Think immune dysfunction, nutritional imbalance, endocrine dysregulation, and/or psychological stressors? If it is one or all, it is where we start.

Once we optimize the patient's endocrine function (see thyroid/HPA section) and lifestyle/nutritional changes have been made, we ought to consider the other etiologies of fatigue. Reflect on the history. This is where an excellent questionnaire will come into play. Rule out other basic possible causes of fatigue: thyroid, depression, and so on. If the history lends itself to possible infectious etiology "had mono ... never recovered" or "my glands swell here and there and then I suffer with bouts of fatigue ... worse than my other fatigue," then consider CFS secondary to infectious etiology.

EBV and cytomegalovirus Immunoglobulin M (CMV IgM) as well as IgG antibodies should be checked and used as a guide. Leading CFS researcher, Dr. Jose Montoya, recommends checking EBV, CMV titres. Several cytokines were found to be elevated in Dr. Montoya's research; furthermore, when they separated the research subjects into mild, moderate, and severe, they reported clinically significant, directly correlated, increases in inflammatory cytokines.[27] I suggest also testing genetics, in my experience, a SOD2 SNP. I always think mitochondrial insufficiency.[28]

ATP is our energy, and mitochondria are our powerhouses. Tying into this mitochondrial/ATP connection is nutrient deficiencies, especially those related to the Krebs and tricarboxylic acid cycle (TCA) cycle. Studies have shown that concentrations of organic acids related to

---

[27] https://med.stanford.edu/news/all-news/2017/07/researchers-id-biomarkers-associated-withchronic-fatigue-syndrome.html.

[28] V. A. Ahmetov, A. E. Naumov, A. Donnikov, E. S. Maciejewska-Karłowska, A. K. Kostryukova, and Larin, "*SOD2* gene polymorphism and muscle damage markers in elite athletes," *Free Radic Res* (Jun 23, 2014): 948–955, DOI: 10.3109/10715762.2014.928410.

the TCA cycle and energy metabolism, such as citrate, isocitrate, and malate, are significantly lower in CFS patients, thus suggesting and supporting the likelihood of less than optimal ATP output.[29]

The Krebs cycle nutrient requirements include many specific vitamins and minerals to help metabolize fats, carbohydrates, and protein to create energy. If you can do a panel inclusive of all fat- and water-soluble nutrient metabolites, amino acids, and antioxidants, then by all means, do. If limited by resources or need to be conscious of patient cost, I suggest you test a serum CoQ10, RBC glutathione, RBC magnesium, and manganese, and if you are able, add vitamins B1, B2, and B3. Also important to note, some people have genetic mutations of NQO1, which, if abnormal, may impede the conversion of CoQ10 into ubiquinol.[30]

> **Fast Fact**
>
> What does B1 (thiamine) have to do with energy? Pyruvate dehydrogenase complex generates the acetyl CoA that enters the Krebs cycle (ATP production and oxidation of fats, protein, and carbohydrates), and one of the important cofactors necessary for the activity of the pyruvate dehydrogenase complex is thiamine pyrophosphate.

Please do not take the "little is good; more must be better" attitude! Some metabolite testing is available and a nice reference for average total availability. Remember though, metabolic chemical processes are fluctuating moment to moment. All stressors and required metabolic demands will utilize nutrients in many ways—upregulation, downregulation, and so forth—to allow optimal biochemistry to

---

[29] E. Yamano, M. Sugimoto, A. Hirayama, S. Kume, M. Yamato, and G. Jin, and Y. Kataoka, "Index markers of chronic fatigue syndrome with dysfunction of TCA and urea cycles," *Scientific Reports* 6 (34990)(2016), https://doi.org/10.1038/srep34990.

[30] Alexandra Fischer, et al., ". Association between genetic variants in the Coenzyme Q10 metabolism and Coenzyme Q10 status in humans," *BMC Res Notes* 4(2011): 245, DOI: 10.1186/1756-0500-4-245.

achieve homeostasis. However, I do appreciate the testing as a guideline for generalized interpretation of deficiencies versus excesses.

Often, I hear the argument, "Supplementation is not necessary." My answer is this: If the specimen in study is healthy, has no genetic mutations that interfere with optimal biochemical pathway function, is under no excessive lengthy stress (sleeping adequately, rising with the sun, and sleeping at dark), eating a balanced seasonal plant-based (including grass-fed meat) diet from plants grown in healthy nutrient-rich soil, and is enjoying community and receiving daily love, then yes, I agree that person would not tend to need extra nutrient supplementation.

However, I imagine we would be hard-pressed to find patients who would fill that description. Thus, my motto is "replace when needed, first with food, and less is best!" (The least dose and number of supplements is the wisest choice for compliance and your patient's pocketbook.) In summary, mitochondrial ATP optimization is key for all bodily functions, including elimination, biotransformation, and immune and endocrine regulation, to name a few.

The second step is to look for causes of depletion, like stress (acute or chronic illness, lifestyle, diet, exogenous toxicity exposures, etc.) This investigation could include blood, urine, and hair testing as well as a great history. Test for infectious causes if history lends or if there is no improvement with the first recommendation. If their story directs you to possible environmental exposures, for instance, chemicals, heavy metals, poly pharmacy, mold, and so forth, then consider testing for this.

My experience has taught me a very fundamental application. If given the basic required nutrients and you remove the exposure, the body is smarter than I ever will be and will optimize function without much intervention. As a clinician, my advice is to support the system and give it time.

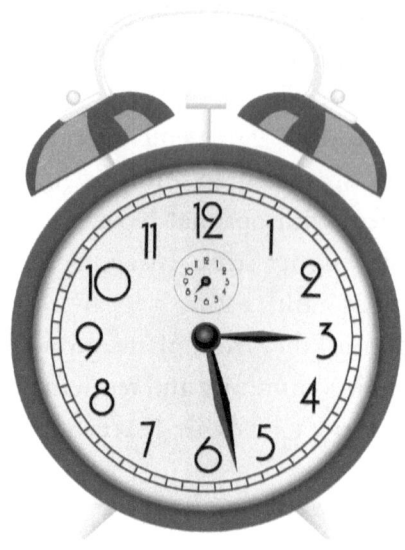

TIME

How long will it be until I am better doctor? This is where individuality comes into play. Treat the patient and be attentive to their presentation. Adjust treatment and support frequently and as needed. Do not treat the lab. And no one is textbook.

This is as good place as any to mention why I feel frequent treatment adjustments make huge differences. Often the best outcomes I have had, usually with the most difficult (health challenges or otherwise) patients, were when I had to listen to their story once to get the base and then again when a new symptom evolved and then again and again if necessary.

> Like a good investigator, I read once all the way through to get the main point and then take it piece by piece. Each presentation is like a new chapter, all a process in their healing. As I learn more, I adjust my treatment and recommendations accordingly.

The amount of time it takes, of course, depends on what type of infection the patient is experiencing. Elevated IgM titres for EBV, parvovirus, or CMV are indicative of an acute infection; nonetheless the elevated IgG results can mean a chronic ongoing viral response. As stated in a respected research publication, *World Journal of Virology*,

> Immunocompetent patients, cytotoxic T lymphocytes and NK cells control the growth of transformed cells during primary infection, particularly the CD8+ T cells directed against antigens of the lytic cycle.[31] These cells are also directed against antigens of the latent phase, but the response is insufficient to ensure their complete

---

[31] Luke R. Williams, Laura L. Quinn, Martin Rowe, and K. Jianmin Zuo, "Pathogenesis and Immunity-Induction of the Lytic Cycle Sensitizes Epstein-Barr Virus-Infected B Cells to NK Cell Killing That Is Counteracted by Virus-Mediated NK Cell Evasion Mechanisms in the Late Lytic Cycle," Journal of Virology (Nov. 10, 2015), DOI: 10.1128/JVI.01932-15.

eradication, and the virus can persist throughout life with low or intermittent levels of virion production.[32],[33]

This constant immune battle may result in nutrient depletion, endocrine dysfunction (e.g., disrupting thyroid conversion), and ultimately, as a result of elevated oxidative stress, alter DNA.[34] Scientific research of post-transplant patients in 2012 confirmed type-III latency of infectious mononucleosis and chronic/active EBV infection (EBNA1, -2, -3A, -3B, -3C; LMP1, LMP2, EBERs, BARTs) can result in lymphoproliferative disorders, AIDS-related immunoblastic illness, or brain lymphoma.

The following is an interpretation of EBV serological profiles in immunocompetent patients:

Anti-EBV antibodies			Interpretation
VCA IgM	VCA IgG	EBNA-1 IgG	
Negative	Negative	Negative	No immunity
Positive	Negative	Negative	Acute infection or non-specificity[1]

---

[32] Q. Y. Yao, A. B. Rickinson, and M. A. Epstein, "A re-examination of the Epstein-Barr virus carrier state in healthy seropositive individuals," *Int J Cancer* 35(1985): 35–42, PMID: 2981780, DOI:10.1002/ijc.2910350107.

[33] M. De Paschale and C. Pierangelo, "Serological diagnosis of Epstein-Barr virus infection: Problems and Solutions," *World J Virol* 1(1)(2012): 31–43, DOI: 10.5501/wjv.v1.i1.31.

[34] Ilaria Liguori, Gennaro Russo, Francesco Curcio, Giulia Bulli, Luisa Aran, David Della-Morte, Gaetano Gargiulo, Gianluca Testa, Francesco Cacciatore, Domenico Bonaduce, and Pasquale Abete, "Oxidative stress, aging, and diseases," *Clin Interventional Aging* 13(2018): 757–772, DOI: 10.2147/CIA.S158513, PMCID: PMC5927356, PMID: 29731617.

Positive	Positive	Negative	Acute infection
Negative	Positive	Positive	Past infection
Negative	Positive	Negative	Acute or past infection[1]
Positive	Positive	Positive	Late primary infection or reactivation[1]
Negative	Negative	Positive	Past infection or non-specificity[1]

No wonder why they might be tired! So what can we do?

First, use meditation, but not the "slow your thoughts, sit on a pillow, light a candle, and hum like a yogi" kind of mindfulness. Use something like the Ziva technique (which I found that I like) that helps truly lower your sympathetic activity at least twenty minutes per day, ideally fifteen minutes twice per day. Variable heart rate monitors are helpful tools for patients as well. I like the HeartMath tool. Regardless of the technique or tools, this is not an option. For some, a nap around 1:30 to 3:00 p.m. is best. Trying to lower high cortisol states and matching a healthier circadian rhythm is my goal.

As for exercise, I have long said "exercise may be your stress reliever," but it still raises a fight-or-flight cascade of hormones, which is not helpful if you are already exhausted and your reserves are low. (Exercise is very important. In fatigued patients, I only allow mindful walking at first and then advancing exercise eventually and slowly.)

Though we have been taught CFS (fibromyalgia as well) patients need to exercise, when they are so tired they can barely get showered and dressed to come see you, they do not have the reserves for exercise. It is true: exercise increases mitochondrial production, but in the immediate state of severe fatigue, the amount of oxidative stress created with even a short burst of exercise still requires increased ATP, thus increased demand on nutrient stores, especially antioxidants.

Along with nutrient optimization, I recommend treating the viral load. There are several theories. Is this truly a high chronic antigenic infection, or is the body reacting chronically to what was once an active viral infection? No one is sure as of 2019. Either way, clinically reducing the patient's infectious load most often results in happier, more energetic patients. Whether you opt for herbal antiviral/bacterial/fungal or medicinal as your preferential treatment will depend on your training. Nevertheless, I use both.[35]

I have another tip: herbal treatments alter biochemistry just as prescription medicine does, but none are without adverse reactions. Some of my favorite herbal support for viral etiologies include olive leaf, Ocimum basilicum (sweet basil), cat's claw, and garlic. For bacterial support, try Berberine, Oregon grape, goldenseal, garlic, or Coptis chinesis. For fungal support, try Pau d'arco, garlic, oregano, Berberine, or ginger.

The key for proper treatment selection, as with any diagnosis in medicine, is to do a proper history and workup so you can narrow your differential diagnosis. I endorse frequent assessments of the patient's clinical response. Once you feel you are or have addressed the trigger/mediator adequately, it is time to rebuild.

For the final and considered my third step, slowly increase your patient's exercise demand, increase their ATP support nutritionally, and slowly decrease the infectious treatments. Assess often (even with a quick nurse check-in).

All in all, for patients with a pathogenic chronic fatigue syndrome/ME diagnosis, I hope you will consider a functional medicine approach.

---

[35] Of note, for the purpose of this book, I will not include parasite/amoebic infections, though they do exist.

Simple alterations in lifestyle and basic foundational repair (including nutrient support and optimal biochemistry), ultimately followed by pertinent treatment of infectious etiologies, will prove to be rewarding for both your patient and you.

CHAPTER FOUR

AUTOIMMUNE DISORDERS

Autoimmune disorders following on the tail of the CFS section seems appropriate. Most patients I have encountered with autoimmune disease also suffer from above average fatigue, though not true ME. Autoimmune disease is complex, and often patients have several diagnoses.

ANTINUCLEAR ANTIBODIES (ANA) POSITIVE AND REFLEX ANTIBODY NEGATIVE

Doctors, how often have you told your patients the following: "This is okay," "It does not mean you have an autoimmune disease," "It is merely a screening tool," or "We will continue to follow your labs, and I will refer you to rheumatologist if you present with a cohort of symptoms and/or your titers are above XYZ"?

New science has demonstrated this old "you have the gene so you will get the disease" model is wrong.

> If a patient has a genetic predisposition/strong family history of an autoimmune disorder and an ANA screening antibody low positive (AKA borderline) presents to your office, remember that this doesn't guarantee an autoimmune disorder, but if environmental conditions turn that process on and are not ceased, then statistics suggest a chronic autoimmune disease in later life.

As a clinician, I gain incredible satisfaction by successfully preventing such fate. It goes without saying: of course, it makes for a fulfilling job when you can slow the progression of active disease! Just think early intervention!

Biologics and immune-modulating medications are important and very effective, but my goal is the same for all dysfunctions. Let us use the least number of pharmaceuticals needed to achieve benefit and ultimately improve quality of life.

Would it not be wonderful to put some control in the hands of our patients and even money in their pockets? The cost of disease-modifying antirheumatic drugs (DMARDS) and biologics (medicine for autoimmune disorders) are anywhere from $100 to $3,000 per month, depending on the frequency and the newness of the drug. Nevertheless, the exciting progress of new biologics also equates to an increase in prescription costs for patients.

A second consequence of many autoimmune diseases are the costly interventions needed because of bodily damage caused by the inflammatory process of the disease. For instance, most surgeries related to rheumatoid arthritis are joint replacements, which cost tens of thousands of dollars. Astoundingly, the average cost of a total knee replacement surgery in the United States in 2018 was approximately $31,000.[1] Recent research suggests 50 percent of patients with rheumatoid arthritis become unable to work within ten years of disease onset.[36]

And the overall cost of treating autoimmune disease in the United States, according to the National Institutes of Allergy and Infectious Diseases (NIAID,) has estimated it to be greater than $100 billion annually. Current recommendations are not to watch and wait, but early intervention once you have established a diagnosis.

---

[36] E. M. Barrett, D. G. I. Scott, N. J. Wiles, and D. P. M. Symmons, "The impact of rheumatoid arthritis on employment status in the early years of disease: a UK community-based study," *Rheumatology* 39(12)(2000): 1403–1409, https://doi.org/10.1093/rheumatology/39.12.1403.

Fast Fact (Not So Fun in This Case)

Patients with autoimmune disorders, such as rheumatoid arthritis, have at least a 50 percent risk of mortality from cardiovascular disease, especially ischemic events, and to top that off, the risk of developing heart disease is 48 to 70 percent above a patient without rheumatoid arthritis.[37,38]

Rheumatoid arthritis controlled with DMARDs and biologics decrease the risk, especially if the patient follows a healthier lifestyle and controls other risk factors such as blood pressure and cholesterol. However, it should be noted the DMARDS and biologics have proven to increase cholesterol, a catch twenty-two in this case![39]

Key Point

Prescription medicine is not the evil here; ideally work to achieve homeostasis and complement the necessary prescriptions.

However, before implementation of the standard of care, one must have a diagnosis driven by fulminant symptoms and usually strong positive lab tests. Functional medicine application is a way we can step in even earlier.

---

[37] Thomas Zegkos, George Kitas, and Theodoros Dimitroulas "Cardiovascular risk in rheumatoid arthritis: assessment, management and next steps," *Ther Adv Musculoskeletal Dis* 8(3)(2016): 86–101, DOI:10.1177/1759720X16643340, PMCID: PMC4872174.

[38] Christina Charles-Schoeman, MD, MS, "Cardiovascular Disease and Rheumatoid Arthritis: An Update," *Curr Rheumatol Rep* 14(5)(2012): 455–462, DOI: 10.1007/s11926-012-0271-5, PMCID: PMC3436948, NIHMSID: NIHMS393529, PMID: 22791398.

[39] Rishi J. Desai, MS, PhD, Wesley Eddings, PhD, Katherine P Liao, MD, MPH, Daniel H Solomon, MD, MPH, and Seoyoung C Kim, MD ScD MSCE, "Disease modifying anti-rheumatic drug use and the risk of incident hyperlipidemia in patients with early rheumatoid arthritis: A retrospective cohort study," *Arthritis Care Res (Hoboken)* 67(4)(2015): 457–466, DOI: 10.1002/acr.22483, PMCID: PMC4751079, NIHMSID: NIHMS634440, PMID: 25302481.

HOW MIGHT YOU DO THIS?

Essentially look for all possible underlying inflammatory stimulants. Then control them and support proper immune function. And of course, if needed, use medication, but optimize supporting pathways and nutrients to ward off side effects and adverse reactions. I will not target specific autoimmune disorders in this chapter because it has been my experience this primary care functional medicine approach is applicable to all autoimmune presentations with equally positive results.

Let's break it down. I find a simple analogy helps.

Let's say the autoimmune disease is the fire, whether it is a raging forest fire or a smoldering coal pit. At a minimum, we should do our best to calm the fire. Identifying several areas of action follows our detection of an ongoing inflammatory process. These are the dependent variables. I explain it to the patient as" fuel being poured on the fire." The more fuel we have, the hotter the fire will burn. And if I can identify and stop "multiple canisters of lighter fluid from pouring onto their raging fire," then we can decrease the symptoms and damage.

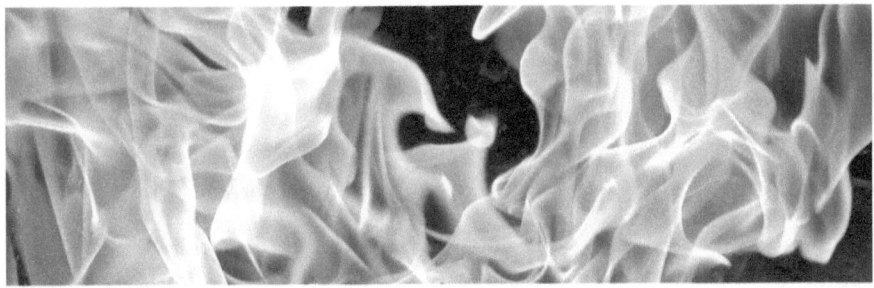

PUT OUT THE FIRE!

This is key for all disease processes, not just autoimmune diseases.

> Applying the basic functional medicine principles allows practitioners to identify and rectify the imbalance. Utilize the matrix to pinpoint the trigger(s) and/or mediator(s) for the autoimmune dysregulation.

An imperative focus should be on proper GI function. The research literature in the last ten years has been flooded with the discovery of the relative relationship the gastrointestinal tract has with the immune system.[40],[41] Assure your patient has proper daily bowel movements and good gastrointestinal mucosal health. You can test this with a comprehensive stool analysis, ideally one that is inclusive of commensal microbiome polymerase chain reaction (PCR) testing and inflammatory assessments, fecal sIgA especially. And of course, treat any pathogens not common in the gastrointestinal tract.

Glutamine and zinc have shown to be beneficial to mucosal health. Incorporating these nutrients proves helpful in most patients in my practice. I also emphasize the appropriate eating plan for the individual, and if able, incorporate probiotic foods as much as possible to assure a healthy microbiome, another key treatment in my practice.[42]

In summary, first identify areas of potential inflammation. You should investigate diet, stress, poor sleep, optimized assimilation and digestion, infection (dental, EBV, herpes simplex virus [HSV], human

---

[40] Yasmine Belkaid and Timothy Hand, "Role of the Microbiota in Immunity and inflammation," *Cell* 157(1)(2014): 121–141, DOI: 10.1016/j.cell.2014.03.011, PMCID: PMC4056765, NIHMSID: NIHMS579635, PMID: 24679531.

[41] Veronica Lazar, Lia-Mara Ditu, Gratiela Gradisteanu Pircalabioru, Irina Gheorghe, Carmen Curutiu, Alina Maria Holban, Ariana Picu, Laura Petcu, and Mariana Carmen Chifiriuc, "Aspects of Gut Microbiota and Immune System Interactions in Infectious Diseases, Immunopathology, and Cancer," *Front Immunol* (August 15, 2018), https://doi.org/10.3389/fimmu.2018.01830.

[42] Blaise CorthésyMulti-Faceted Functions of Secretory IgA at Mucosal Surfaces," *Front Immunol* 4(2013): 185, DOI: 10.3389/fimmu.2013.00185, PMCID: PMC3709412, PMID: 23874333.

papillomavirus [HPV], etc.), and toxins. Second and most importantly, with the tips in this book, eliminate or at least decrease these drivers. Then do your best to work as a team and empower the patient to maintain their new healthy lifestyle.

CHAPTER FIVE

THYROID: "THE MASTER GLAND"

THYROID

The thyroid is a large controller of the hypothalamus and pituitary feedback loop. It is often spoken of as the master gland (an oversimplification, in my opinion), but it's an important endocrine organ nonetheless. Because it is a regulator of our metabolism, temperature, and many other systems, I feel optimal function of this gland is a "bang for buck." Ideal function allows for better regulation of weight, temperature, immune function, and, indirectly, better mood and cognition, to mention a few.

As we were taught in medical training, check TSH. If it is greater than 5.0 (10.0 not too long ago), then treat the hypothyroid. This is problematic because TSH is just that, a hormone produced to signal the thyroid to increase or decrease the production of thyroid hormone. Let us refresh our memory in a shortened version: The pituitary stimulates the thyroid, which produces T4 (inactive). T4 is then converted into free T3 (fT3), described as the "accelerator" in my practice. Reverse T3 (rT3), is "the parking brake."

Most of the literature suggests that the conversion of fT3 to rT3 is a 50/50 ratio; though this is when all is in balance, as in the hypothalamic–pituitary–adrenal (HPA) axis is not dysfunctional. Therefore, if you have good intentions of optimizing thyroid function, you must instill some HPA lifestyle support as well.

One must always consider this for the patient who presents with an illness (chronic or acute), never sleeps, and lives on caffeine (an extended high sympathetic state) because they may very well have high cortisol and/or catecholamines. This high sympathetic hormonal cascade influences the negative feedback loop to slow the patient down. Their body is encouraging rest by increasing rT3 and decreasing gonadal output, among other things.[43]

Fun Fact

Mildly increased serum TSH (4.5–9.9 mIU/L) is associated with diastolic dysfunction, dyslipidemia, and vascular alterations in young and middle-aged patients.[1, 2] These adverse effects improved after replacement therapy with L-thyroxine in randomized controlled studies.[1, 2]

TSH

⇕

T4 (inactive) ←● T3
("accelerator"): rT3("brake")

+Cortisol, NE ⇕

Gonadal hormones

TSH●FT4●FT3

TG⤴   ⤴TPO

---

[43] Wang, Appendix B (2018).

It is fair to reason, if you falsely increase free t3 or free t4 while the body is sending signals to slow down, the patient will feel good for a couple of days (e.g., more energy, better sense of calm, and improved sleep), but then the miraculous body overrides your attempts to upregulate their endocrine system. The patient, who was for a moment singing your praises, is now calling your office, reporting to your staff that they are worse! Exhausted! They cannot function. The parking brake is now on full force!

This is the beauty of functional medicine. It ideally starts with lifestyle, commonsense basics, first. I will circle back to this because ideal is often not real-life, practical implication. Nevertheless, I recommend you have had a chat with your patient on initial presentation, following the "I'm tired, I think it's my thyroid, and on the Google checklist I'm checking boxes left and right, doc" comment.

At this point, implementing daily deep breathing, regular naps (short power naps), and/or quiet time would be of upmost importance. Also adding in a diet that is supportive of thyroid health and foods that increase serotonin and help lower cortisol and insulin should be their new dietary focus.

After two to three weeks of this habit installation, they should return and have thyroid levels checked and compared to their initial levels. What has changed? Usually in my experience, the conversion of free T4 to free T3 has improved and the rt3 is lower.

If not and you find rT3 is high, free is T4 low, and T3 is low-normal, it's time to give them a little boost, a little help in the right direction. A low-dose t4 replacement is one of your first options. Remember, your reference range for normal (my recommendation is always safe practice) above 1 ng/dl is recommended by most or above the middle average of the lab normal reference range. (Most laboratory reference ranges are 0.8–2.5ng/dl).[44]

> **Fast Fact**
>
> Have you ever wondered how we get normal values for laboratory ranges? Reference ranges are based on average normals of healthy individuals and what average units are seen most in a lab at a given time. Laboratory normal values can be changed based on what they see over time.

Keep that in mind when someone encourages you to treat a patient only based on a lab value.

As long as their thyroid conversation is not impeded, then a small amount of t4, inactive thyroid, replacement will help increase free t3 "the go juice" (accelerator), as I call it, and if they are applying the lifestyle changes you recommended for them at their first visit, their innate "parking brake" (rt3), will not slam on in response to the increased thyroid activity.

Thyroid conversion is important to consider when? Always! The easiest way to discern who may be a poor converter is to ask. Get a family history and review past medical records. I cannot tell you how often I have found abnormal labs but no treatment was given because TSH was normal.

With a history of Hashimoto's or autoimmune thyroiditis or personal or family history, odds are they will have had a lab abnormality of either Thyroglobulin (TG) or Thyroid peroxidase (TPO) antibodies, if you

---

[44] Begoña Ruiz-Núñez, Rabab Tarasse, Emar F. Vogelaar, D. A. Janneke Dijck-Brouwer, and A. J. Frits, "Higher Prevalence of "Low T3 Syndrome" in Patients With Chronic Fatigue Syndrome: A Case-Control Study," *Frontiers of Endocrinology* 9(2018): 97, DOI: 10.3389/fendo.2018.00097, PMCID: PMC5869352, PMID: 29615976.

see poor conversion. If you see abnormal conversion (normal free t4 and low t3 with normal rT3 and no antibodies), please keep in mind genetic polymorphisms. DIO and TSHR variants create poorer thyroid hormone production, conversion, and uptake in the cells.[45] (There are a couple more antibodies, but we are sticking to the basics here. Refer to endocrinology otherwise.)

Let's review the microsomal enzyme (TPO) and thyroglobulin (TG) enzyme purpose. It's a must know to understand the pathophysiology. It's nothing medical school did not teach us. It's just important to review.

Thyroglobulin is an important protein in the thyroid because it is required to produce thyroxine and triiodothyronine.

$$TSH > FT4 \rightarrow \rightarrow \rightarrow FT3$$

$$TG\uparrow \quad \uparrow TPO$$

TPO enzyme is important for the inactive t4 hormone conversion to the active t3 hormone. If you have high antibody activity toward either of these, your body's ability to function optimally from a thyroid standpoint is impaired. For example, the person with high TPO antibodies has an immune system that attacks this enzyme. Simply put, it is no longer available to convert the levothyroxine (T4) you have prescribed them into the active thyroid hormone. It doesn't matter how much thyroid medicine (t4) you give them. If the body is dysregulated, it will make more antibodies (a stranger-danger reaction from the immune system). In response, your patient will feel just as tired, if not more.

How many patients have you looked at and either shrugged or felt helpless after they returned from a hopeful office visit where you both

---

[45] E. Park, J. Jung, O. Araki, et al., "Concurrent TSHR mutations and DIO2 T92A polymorphism result in abnormal thyroid hormone metabolism," Sci Rep 8(10090) (July 2018), DOI:10.1038/s41598-018-28480-0.

were sure a little thyroid medicine would help them feel better? Now, they sit there looking at you as if you stole their favorite stuffed animal.

In this scenario of Hashimoto's (high TPO, AKA microsomal antibodies), my suggestion is to add a bit of t3 (liothyronine) and then recheck in four to six weeks and assure TSH, free t4, and free t3 remain in normal range. Don't forget: we must also do all we can to help the conversion process. Much help should come from a healthy diet and anything else we know to do to calm the immune response, especially if an autoimmune disorder is active or present. For example, vitamin D is necessary for proper conversion. Trace iodine, zinc, and selenium also play a role. If you don't know what foods are high in these nutrients, then consult a trained dietitian. (See my list at the end of the book for personal references.)

Optimizing vitamin D levels is imperative and important in several metabolic processes. Vitamin D is a hormone that is necessary for thyroid conversion version and immune regulation. Thus, in reference to proper thyroid function, check a vitamin D 25-hydroxy level, and shoot for an optimal range of 50 to 70 ng/mL. Some will say vitamin D levels could and should be higher; however, there is literature that suggests levels higher than 70 ng/mL can cause some calcium displacement from the bones. "Vitamin D toxicity is associated with enhanced re-absorption of bone in some patients."[46] To err on the side of caution, I recommend practitioners to stick to 50 to 60 ng/mL.

Checking the patient's nutrient deficiencies is, of course, a spot check, as nutrient requirements change and many cellular shifts occur throughout the day. (Thus, vitamin and mineral levels will change and fluctuate throughout the day.) However, a lab test for nutrient deficiencies does give you a baseline to reference and make suggestions.

---

[46] Hansen KE. High-dose vitamin D: helpful or harmful? Curr Rheumatol Rep. 2011;13(3):257–264. doi:10.1007/s11926-011-0175-9

Something to remember: a lot of your nutrient requirements are micronutrients, particularly most minerals. Tiny amounts for replacement are usually all that is necessary. For example, when replacing iodine, it's much safer and easier as food replacement. Having someone eat seaweed regularly or Brazil nuts is an excellent way of increasing their iodine and selenium. If you want to replace iodine with a supplement, then I recommend you check a serum iodine or a urine iodine. It is a common deficiency throughout the world, as 9 percent of the Americas are deficient according to *Lancet* 2003.[47]

Frequently clinicians ask how often they must check the thyroid, and I believe is it imperative to check the entire thyroid panel after the initial assessment. I check the entire panel—as in TSH, free T3, and free T4—four to six weeks after I start replacement, sooner if needed, and again six weeks later to see if we are maintaining a normal range. Then it's once or twice per year. Have the patient come back into the office to assess their clinical response and then check TSH once or twice a year as needed.

The key is to educate your patients to be an active participant in their health care and be aware of the side effects of taking thyroid replacement, especially if they're taking too much. A TSH result in the hyper range should also be followed with a bone density scan every couple of years. I've never had a patient have osteopenia or osteoporosis as a result of treatment in this manner. Before you start treatment, do a baseline bone density if you're concerned. After a clinical trial of approximately three months, if the patient has not had noticeable improvement, then stop

---

[47] Bruno de Benoist, Maria Andersson, Bahi Takkouche, and Ines Egli, "Prevalence of iodine deficiency worldwide," *Lancet* (November 29, 2003), DOI: https://doi.org/10.1016/S0140-6736(03)14920-3.
My clinical experience has shown that several people feel very good with the TSH level that is slightly in the "hyper range." If free T4 and free T3 are normal, then I document that as a euthyroid response and confirm the patient is having no hyper thyroid symptoms.

the medicine and continue your investigation. Continue the lifestyle modifications!

The literature is overflowing with data informing practitioners of the perils of thyroid replacement when not necessary, especially t3. Not all will benefit.[48] Nevertheless, there are an equal amount of resources referencing the variation in conditions and the patient populations that could benefit from individualized thyroid replacement, and more research is needed in this area.

Flaws in experimental design from most randomized controlled trials on this subject have produced ambiguous results that lack physiological, individualized biochemistry. By deductive reasoning and experience in research, I must consider the lack of funding, driven by a lack of pharmaceutical interest, as a limiting factor for the deficiency of such research, but we can hope.

Fast Fact

The most recent American Association of Clinical Endocrinologists (AACE) and American Thyroid Association (ATA) guidelines support treatment of mild subclinical hypothyroidism in patients with evidence of atherosclerotic cardiovascular disease and heart failure or in the presence of risk factors associated with these disorders.[49]

---

[48] A. Pingitore, E. Galli, A. Barison, A. Iervasi, M. Scarlattini, D. Nucci, A. L'abbate, R. Mariotti, and G. Iervasi, "Acute effects of triiodothyronine (T3) replacement therapy in patients with chronic heart failure and low-T3 syndrome: a randomized, placebo-controlled study," *J Clin Endocrinol Metab* 93(4)(2008): 1351–1358, DOI: 10.1210/jc.2007-2210.

[49] J. C. Nelson and R. T. Tomei, "Direct determination of free thyroxin in undiluted serum by equilibrium dialysis/radioimmunoassay," *Clin Chem* 34(1988): 1737–1744, PMID: 3138040.

My intention here is to help the provider consider all information as they assess their patient individually. Let the labs and randomized controlled trials be a guide but not an end-all, definitive plan of action. Thyroid function is a subject that needs more research, and in the meantime, err on the side of caution, treat the patient, and utilize all information to guide your decisions and document!

Thyroid assessment and proper treatment is clearly more than checking a TSH, as that is an antiquated approach. Consider your patient's genetics and full pathophysiological testing and listen to them. Proper treatment will result in happy patients and healthier populations.

CHAPTER SIX

VITAMIN D

In the last five years, I learned I have a few vitamin D receptor (VDR) polymorphisms (genetic mutation), which interferes with the uptake of vitamin D into the cell. I recall when I started vitamin D in 2009. At high doses, my skin rash improved.

Vitamin D is vital for immune regulation and an excellent area of action for inflammatory disorders, making optimization especially important in all autoimmune disorders, brain and bone health, and even mental health. This is, in my opinion, where an area PCPs can easily make an impact.

It has been known for more than twenty years that vitamin D exerts marked effects on immune, DNA/RNA, and even neuronal cells. These nonclassical actions of vitamin D have recently gained a renewed attention since it has been shown that diminished levels of vitamin D induce immune-mediated symptoms in animal models of autoimmune diseases and is a risk factor for various brain diseases.

For example, in 2017, research demonstrated that vitamin D "modulates the production of several neurotrophins, up-regulates Interleukin-4 and inhibits the differentiation and survival of dendritic cells, resulting in impaired allo-reactive T cell activation."[50] Not surprisingly, vitamin D has been found to be a strong risk-modifying factor for multiple sclerosis (MS), the most prevalent neurological and inflammatory disease in the young adult population.

We all know the relationship between vitamin D and bone health, including osteoporosis, osteopenia, and osteomalacia. Vitamin D deficiency is more common than we think, and though some say it is a concern, others think it is a pandemic. Either way, I feel vitamin D, with its many hormonal purposes, is one of those low-hanging fruits, which, when necessary, we can optimize and assist in functional restoration.

Vitamin D is a secosteroid hormone, produced photochemically in the animal epidermis. The action of ultraviolet light (UVB) on 7-dehydrocholesterol results in the production of pre-vitamin D, which, after thermoconversion and two separate hydroxylations, gives rise to the active 1,25-dihydroxyvitamin D.

It is important to understand genetic polymorphisms, age, skin color, and, of course, diet and activity levels are among the many factors playing a role in a patient's serum level.[51,52] Vitamin D acts through two types of receptors: (i) the VDR, a member of the steroid/thyroid hormone superfamily of transcription factors, and (ii) the membrane associated, rapid response steroid binding (MARRS) receptor, also known as Erp57/Grp58.

---

[50] D. A. Fernandes de Abreu, D. Eyles, and F. Féron, "Vitamin D, a neuro-immunomodulator: implications for neurodegenerative and autoimmune diseases," *Psychoneuroendocrinology* 34 Suppl 1(2009): S265–77, DOI: 10.1016.

[51] Zhu Haidong, Jigar Bhagatwala, Ying Huang, Norman K. Pollock, Samip Parikh, Anas Raed, Bernard Gutin, Gregory A. Harshfield, and Yanbin Dong, "Race/Ethnicity-Specific Association of Vitamin D and Global DNA Methylation: Cross-Sectional and Interventional Findings," *PLoS One* 11(4)(2016): e0152849, DOI: 10.1371/journal.pone.0152849, PMCID: PMC4822838, PMID: 27049643.

[52] J. Christopher Gallagher, MD, MRCP, "Vitamin D and Aging," *Endocrinol Metab Clin North Am* 42(2)(2013): 319–332, doi: 10.1016/j.ecl.2013.02.004, PMCID: PMC3782116, NIHMSID: NIHMS46644, PMID: 23702404.

Common SNP is the VDR mutation, making it difficult for patients with this mutation to transport vitamin D into cells. It is my experience these patients will have elevated serum 26 hydroxy-vitamin D levels with supplementation but quickly drop when supplementation is ceased. I have found it to be best if I keep my patients with VDR TaQ mutations on 5,000 IU after I achieve optimal levels, checking levels yearly.

In this 1987 article, Schwartzman reviewed some of the mechanisms that may underlie the role of vitamin D in various brain diseases.

> We then assess how vitamin D imbalance may lay the foundation for a range of adult disorders, including brain pathologies (Parkinson's disease, epilepsy, depression) and immune-mediated disorders (rheumatoid arthritis, type I diabetes mellitus, systemic lupus erythematous or inflammatory bowel diseases).[53]

Multidisciplinary scientific collaborations are now required to fully appreciate the complex role of vitamin D in mammal metabolism, as demonstrated in the 2009 *Psychoneuroendocrinology* publication.[54]

Hypervitaminosis D can cause bone rapid turnover and even increase risk for kidney stones, hypertension, and atherosclerosis, especially as a result of hypercalcemia. I feel it is important to be aware that several prescription medications can increase vitamin D potential, including but not limited to thiazides, estrogen therapy, antacids, and digoxin.

An optimal vitamin D range has not been agreed upon, but safely a range of 50 to 70 ng/mL seems to be optimal without any documented adverse effects. As with everything though, just because a little is good

---

[53] M. S. Schwartzman and W. A. Franck, "Vitamin D toxicity complicating the treatment of senile, postmenopausal, and glucocorticoid-induced osteoporosis. Four case reports and a critical commentary on the use of vitamin D in these disorders," *Am J Med* 82(2)(1987): 224–230, PMID:3812514, DOI: 10.1016/0002-9343(87)90060-x.
[54] See footnote 46.

does not mean more is better. Also, of note, ergocalciferol is not the most bioavailable form. Please only prescribe D3, cholecalciferol.

> **Fun Fact**
>
> Ten to fifteen minutes of whole-body exposure to peak summer sun will generate and release up to 20,000 IU vitamin D-3 into the circulation

For primary care health care providers, I would like to point out a few areas I feel vitamin D can make a difference, both quickly and easily.

Seasonal affective disorder (SAD) is common in global areas with long winter months, and especially when I was working at Cleveland Clinic Center for Functional Medicine, I saw several patients have an improvement in their mental health when their vitamin D levels were optimized. It was very prominent in Ohio, but I must admit that hypo vitamin D has been a consistently observed pattern over the last ten years. If my patient already had low vitamin D levels in the winter (below 50 ng/mL), as the vitamin D levels dropped with less sun exposure, their SAD was exacerbated. I had many patients tell me they felt as though a "light was turned on" after recommendation and implementation of replacement.

During my time practicing in Oklahoma, many patients declared, "My vitamin D level can't be low. I am working in the sun all day!" I admit I was puzzled too. The consistent low results with my patients in a state that had summer heat above 100 degrees Fahrenheit prompted investigation.

For this sun-exposed population of my practice, I learned the low levels were in fact real and likely compounded by the fact, if you live above 25 to 35 degrees North latitude (the majority of the United States), you do not live in an area that has adequate sunshine to convert pro D to

D.⁵⁵ Besides, I would lament, "No one I know is really outside in that heat, and if they are, they are covered in SPF 50." Thus, low vitamin D seems to be the case for most of the world, the majority of the year, especially in the winter.

> **Fun Fact**
> Research also tells us that chronic disease, like diabetes, decreases peripheral conversion of thyroid hormone because of a reduction in D2 expression.⁵⁶

FIBROMYALGIA

Vitamin D may even play a role in muscle pain, not just bone pain. Fibromyalgia patients, in my patient population, tend to be low, as did the study participants in a 2016 article published in *Nutrients*.

Interestingly, I also find most of these patients appear to have VDR receptor polymorphisms.

> Overall, although a cause and effect relationship has not been proven yet, available evidence indicates, that vitamin D is a vital bioregulator of pain pathways involved in FM pathogenesis. ... Hypovitaminosis D may be a risk factor for FM and a way of worsening the symptoms through central and peripheral pathways.

---

⁵⁵ Matthias Wacker and Michael F. Holick, "A global perspective for health," *Dermatoendocrinol* 5(1)(2013): 51–108, PMCID: PMC3897598, PMID: 24494042, DOI: 10.4161/derm.24494.

⁵⁶ Rashmi Mullur, Yan-Yun Liu, and Gregory A. Brent, "Thyroid Hormone Regulation of Metabolism," *Physiol Rev* 94(2)(2014): 355–382, DOI: 10.1152/physrev.00030.2013, PMCID: PMC4044302, PMID: 24692351.

The exact mechanisms however, by which vitamin D may be related with FM remain unclear.[57]

Growing pains (osteomalacia) in children or adults presents as deep bone aches/pain. Check vitamin D 25 OH and 1,25 vitamin D as well as total and free ionized calcium. Replace as needed. As for immune regulation and thyroid connection,[58] I need not say more. The literature is there. Just heed my suggestion to optimize levels and follow clinically.

For me, healthy individuals most often do not need replacement with high doses of vitamin D; nevertheless, assuring levels in the high normal range is a goal for my practice. Chronically and acutely ill patients, the more mature population, and, most always, patients with gastrointestinal challenges (IBD, IBS, reflux, and malabsorption) often require 4,000 IU per day on average.

I do recommend you suggest the patient take vitamin D with vitamin K1/K2 (maybe even K7). A patient can fairly easily increase both vitamin D and K in the diet. Tuna, mushrooms, and eggs are high in vitamin D, and dark greens are the best source of K.

Fast Fact

Sweating from the chest up only can be a presentation of vitamin D deficiency.

It's an easy hormone to replace and measure with awesome health benefits, so for PCPs, I recommend paying attention to this gem.

---

[57] Adriana J. van Ballegooijen, Stefan Pilz, Andreas Tomaschitz, Martin R. Grübler, and Nicolas Verheyen "The Synergistic Interplay between Vitamins D and K for Bone and Cardiovascular Health: A Narrative Review," *Int J Endocrinol* (Sept. 12, 2017), DOI: 10.1155/2017/7454376, PMCID: PMC5613455, PMID: 29138634.

[58] S. Karras, E. Rapti, S. Matsoukas, and K. Kotsa, "Vitamin D in Fibromyalgia: A Causative or Confounding Biological Interplay?" *Nutrients* 8(6)(2016), PubMed #27271665.

ADDITIONAL VITAMIN D RESOURCES

1. Adriana J. van Ballegooijen, et al., "The Synergistic Interplay between Vitamins D and K for Bone and Cardiovascular Health: A Narrative Review," *Int J Endocrinol* (2017): 7454376.
2. M. S. Schwartzman, "Vitamin D toxicity complicating the treatment of senile, postmenopausal, and glucocorticoid-induced osteoporosis. Four case reports and a critical commentary on the use of vitamin D in these disorders," *Am J Med* 82(2)(1987): 224–230. Rashmi Mullur, Yan-Yun Liu, and Gregory A. Brent, "Thyroid Hormone Regulation of Metabolism," *Physiol Rev* 94(2) (2014): 355–382, DOI: 10.1152/physrev.00030.2013, PMCID: PMC4044302, PMID: 24692351.
3. Alessandro Marsili, Ann Marie Zavacki, John W. Harney, and P. Reed Larsen, "Physiological role and regulation of iodothyronine deiodinases: a 2011 update," *J Endocrinol Invest* 34(5)(2011): 395–407, DOI: 10.3275/7615, PMCID: PMC3687787, NIHMSID: NIHMS476393, PMID: 21427525.
4. S. Karras, E. Rapti, S. Matsoukas, and K. Kotsa, "Vitamin D in Fibromyalgia: A Causative or Confounding Biological Interplay?" *Nutrients* 8(6)(2016), PubMed #27271665.

CHAPTER SEVEN

CARDIOMETABOLIC HEALTH (HYPERTENSION, CHOLESTEROL, DIABETES/ INSULIN RESISTANCE)

Luckily this is not an area I was challenged with, but it's a huge disease burden on the health-care economics. With more than a million heart attacks and strokes per year, this results in an average monetary burden of more than $300 billion dollars[59] annually with a family burden that is not able to be quantified. "By 2030, annual direct medical costs associated with cardiovascular diseases are projected to rise to more than $818 billion, while lost productivity costs could exceed $275 billion."[60]

Atherosclerotic cardiovascular disease (ASCVD) includes coronary heart disease (CHD), such as myocardial infarction, angina, and coronary artery stenosis. Cerebrovascular disease includes transient ischemic attack (TIA, often referred to as a mini stroke), ischemic stroke, carotid artery stenosis greater than 50 percent blockage, and peripheral artery disease, such as

---

[59] Barbara Bowman, PhD, director of CDC's Division for Heart Disease and Stroke Prevention
[60] CDC Foundation, "Heart Disease and Stroke Cost America Nearly $1 Billion A Day In Medical Costs, Lost Productivity" (April 29, 2015).

claudication. Also, aortic atherosclerotic disease, such as abdominal aortic aneurysms and descending thoracic aneurysm, makes the list of ASCVD.

CRITERIA FOR ASCVD[61]

Atorvastatin and rosuvastatin are now the preferred statins for primary prevention. Nonfasting lipid panel is now the preferred cholesterol test. Aspirin is recommended for patients ages fifty to fifty-nine if there is at least a 10 percent risk of ASCVD (myocardial infarction or stroke) over ten years.

5.0–7.4 percent 10-year risk of ASCVD (myocardial infarction or stroke): Shared decision making. Consider discussing treatment with a moderate-intensity statin.
7.5–14.9 percent 10-year risk: Shared decision making. Consider treatment with a moderate- to high-intensity statin.
≥ 7.5 percent 10-year risk and diabetes, age 40–75: Initiate or continue moderate-intensity statin. Consider use of high-intensity statin.
Age 40–75 with diabetes and LDL 70–189 mg/dL: initiate or continue moderate intensity statins.
≥ 15 percent 10-year risk: Initiate or continue treatment with a moderate- to high-intensity statin.
LDL ≥ 190 mg/dL

Primary prevention refers to the effort to prevent or delay the onset of ASCVD. Secondary prevention refers to the effort to treat known, clinically significant atherosclerotic disease and to prevent or delay the onset of disease manifestations. I feel functional medicine is key for primary prevention.

It is wise to follow the guidelines set forth for us to practice medicine, and when applied with all the skills of a good functional primary

---

[61] "2019 ACC/AHA Guideline on the Primary Prevention of Cardiovascular Disease: A Report of the American College of Cardiology/American Heart Association Task Force on Clinical Practice Guidelines," *J Am Coll Cardiol* (2019).

physician, you will practice in a safe, gratifying environment until you decide to retire. By definition, guidelines are "a rule or principle that provides guidance to appropriate behavior."[62] I follow them to the best of my ability, but I also know my patients are individuals with their own enviro-genetic-stress-biochemical response. This individuality necessitates a more thorough understanding of the situation.

I must mention a recent systemic review published in *JAMA* (March 2019) reported only "8.5% of cardiovascular guidelines are based on randomized controlled trials" and the rest of the guidelines, that some take as gospel, are based on "much weaker evidence."[63]

So please take a good history, do a great exam, document with excellence, and think through the process. The more you understand what it is you are treating, the better you will serve your patients and the more astounding your patient's results will be.

Guidelines evolve as research reveals more and more information. It is dynamic. I suggest we stay up to date. You do no one, primarily your patients, any good if you do not stay up to date. It may be a shock, but clinical application lags approximately twenty years behind research and published guidelines.

So what are the most recent hypertension management guidelines?

As per the Eighth Joint National Committee (JNC8), if a person is diabetic but less than sixty, then the blood pressure goal is 140/90, and if your patient is older than sixty without kidney disease or diabetes, then their blood pressure should be less than 150/90.

---

[62] "Guideline," https://www.definitions.net/definition/guideline.
[63] A. C. Fanaroff, R. M. Califf, S. Windecker, S. C. Smith Jr., and R. D. Lopes, "Levels of Evidence Supporting American College of Cardiology/American Heart Association and European Society of Cardiology Guidelines, 2008–2018," *JAMA* 19;321(11)(2019): 1069–1080, DOI: 10.1001/jama.2019.1122.

As for treatment, first-line agents for most include ACE inhibitors, calcium-channel blockers, and thiazide diuretics. JNC8 suggests triple therapy with these before adding an alpha or beta blocker. If you are treating a patient with kidney disease and hypertension, regardless of ethnic background, initially or adjunctively, an ACE inhibitor or ARB is recommended to protect the kidneys. Not to add to the complexity, if your patient is greater than seventy-five years old with poor renal function, thiazide diuretics or calcium-channel blockers are acceptable treatments. And last, but not least, for all hypertensive patients, JNC8 recommends the Mediterranean diet and advises all to quit smoking.

Speaking of hypertension, I would like to make note of an important point. Often dismissed is the stage one and two blood pressure readings. So many excuses are accepted because we really do not like giving or hearing bad news. "I was stressed this morning … I drank a pot of coffee … I have white coat syndrome." All are often disclosed as reasons the blood pressure is high in the office. But it is akin to raising children. Keeping secrets is not healthy. Call it what it is, hypertension.

Deliver the news, but be ready because usually my savvy patients will try to convince me.

"I have severe white coat syndrome."

"Well," I must ask, "am I that scary? If coming to see me is so stressful that it makes your blood pressure elevated, what happens when you get really stressed or angry throughout the day? The up and down pressure contributes to the vascular damage of vital organs."

Three to four elevated blood pressures in the office receives the diagnosis, and prevention is key. If explained, patients appreciate the understanding. The time between blood pressure checks gives them time to implement lifestyle changes. Lifestyle modification is still guideline recommendation number one, no matter whose guideline you follow, American Heart Association (AHA), Joint National Committee (JNC), or American

Academy of Family Physicians (AAFP). Remind them that vascular resistance, hypertension, and atherosclerosis contribute to heart failure.

Lifestyle modification is not a trendy expression. It can be a cure, a primary prevention of disease. In November 2018, Dr. Benjamin, AHA president, eloquently stated, "The updated guidelines reinforce the importance of healthy living, lifestyle modification and prevention. They build on the major shift we made in our 2013 cholesterol recommendations to focus on identifying and addressing lifetime risks for cardiovascular disease."[64]

Before I go further with treatment, we should be clear about the guidelines for diagnosis.[65]

Normal: Less than 120/80 mm Hg
Elevated: 120–129/80+ mm Hg
Stage 1 Hypertension: 130–139/80–90 mm Hg
Stage 2 Hypertension: At least 140/at least 90 mm Hg
Hypertensive Crisis: 180+/120+ mm Hg and patients needing prompt changes in their medications
Immediate hospitalization if there are signs of organ damage

First, make sure of course you are checking the blood pressure properly. It seems trivial to say, but you would be surprised how few of us know how to properly take a blood pressure. An accurate blood pressure reading is certainly not one recorded after we have hustled the patient into the room while they are shuffling through the kids' snack bag with a cuff wrapped around four fleece shirts. It's a bit exaggerated, but you know what I mean.

---

[64] "Updated cholesterol guidelines offer more personalized risk assessment, additional treatment options for people at the highest risk," https://newsroom.heart.org/news/updated-cholesterol-guidelines-offer-more-personalized-risk-assessment-additional-treatment-options-for-people-at-the-highest-risk.

[65] "New ACC/AHA High Blood Pressure Guidelines Lower Definition of Hypertension," https://www.acc.org/latest-in-cardiology/articles/2017/11/08/11/47/mon-5pm-bp-guideline-aha-2017.

Once the blood pressure readings have been properly logged and the patient has a diagnosis of high blood pressure or even prehypertension, you should ask yourself, "Why does this patient have a blood pressure reading greater than 130 systolic?"

Etiologies of high blood pressure can range from the neuroendocrine response to high stress or lack of sleep or both. It could be attributed to genetics, poor lifestyle/diet choices, and even include environmental toxin exposure or toxic body burdens. The cause can be one or all or a combination of any. This is important to consider.

What's my advice? Use the matrix to identify your patient's likely etiologies. This is a perfect place to start. Insulin resistance is often the biggest modifiable culprit in my patient population. Prediabetes usually coincides with hypercholesterolemia/hypertriglyceridemia. Lifestyle modification can make a huge impact here. Refer to a dietician, stop simple sugars, reduce simple carb intake, and get moving. For those who do not respond immediately to this simple recipe, consider genetic testing to formulate an individualized plan.

> **Fun Fact**
>
> Vitamin D can help lower plasma renin activity.

CHOLESTEROL

Hypertension is among many etiologies of arterial damage, and this can trigger an endothelial repair requiring cholesterol.

As I have said many times, the value of understanding how it happens, the pathophysiology, of any medical issue is paramount. When treating and diagnosing a patient with hypercholesterolemia or, better yet, discussing prevention, the occurrence of cholesterol on the vessel wall should be understood at least in the most basic, up-to-date physiology.

Dispelling the myth that cholesterol is bad is of first order. It is not bad in itself. (A sustained drop in hormones, increased amount of stress, diet combined with malabsorption and genetics, and inflammation can cause an increase in cholesterol in general.) Cholesterol deposition is a response to endothelial damage or inflammation. The deposits can get bigger over time and become unstable, and this stretching of the vessel wall causes thinning, requiring reinforcement in the form of calcium deposits and inflammatory cytokines to keep things in check or restore the area to its baseline. It is understood that the calcifications, though initially protective, in the long term decrease elasticity, resulting in hardening of the arteries. Thus, it's a redundant but necessary theme. For treatment, start at the cause of inflammation. Atherosclerosis starts in childhood, so intervention is never too early. Lifestyle is key!

KNOW THE STUDIES

The more you know and understand the literature, the better you can utilize the information for better outcomes. A 4S study reviewed over four thousand people and demonstrated a 30 percent decrease in total mortality and a 34 percent decrease in coronary events with simvastatin.[66]

The TEXCAPS study took on over six thousand constituents over five years and found, with pravastatin, a 37 percent drop in coronary events and unstable angina. The LIPID study demonstrated, with the use of

---

[66] "Randomised trial of cholesterol lowering in 4444 patients with coronary heart disease: the Scandinavian Simvastatin Survival Study (4S)," *Lancet* 344(8934)(1994): 1383–1389.
J. R. Downs JR[1], M. Clearfield, S. Weis, E. Whitney, D. R. Shapiro, P. A. Beere, A. Langendorfer, E. A. Stein, W. Kruyer, A. M. Gotto Jr., "Primary prevention of acute coronary events with lovastatin in men and women with average cholesterol levels: results of AFCAPS/TexCAPS. Air Force/Texas Coronary Atherosclerosis Prevention Study," *JAMA* 279(20)(1998): 1615–1622.
The LIPID Study Group, "Long-term effectiveness and safety of pravastatin in 9014 patients with coronary heart disease and average cholesterol concentrations: the LIPID trial follow-up," Volume 359 (9315, P1379-1387)(April 20, 2002), DOI: https://doi.org/10.1016/S0140-6736(02)08351-4.

pravastatin in over nine thousand patients, a 22 percent decrease in total mortality and a 24 percent decrease in death from coronary heart disease over six years.

Advanced lipid panels are a must, in my opinion. The old lipid panel, testing only total cholesterol, high-density lipoprotein (HDL), low-density lipoprotein (LDL), and triglycerides, is limited and misses a large portion of patients with cholesterol dysfunction. I will give a basic review of an advanced lipid panel. I have been using them since 2010 for my patients. The basic lipid panel is useful and will suffice if I am treating cholesterol with a statin already, an inexpensive way to monitor LDL, but if my approach is to prevent the pathogenesis of hypercholesterolemia, I like more information.

When I started using them, my colleagues chastised me for this approach: "unnecessary testing and trivial results," "No reason to test when there is nothing you can prescribe them," and "This is experimental and confusing for the patient; plus it adds time to the visit." These were some of the comments I heard, as I defended my reasoning of preventive functional testing. In all fairness I should mention the AHA and American Cardiology Association last statement from 2015. As far as I am aware, they still back the standard cholesterol test.

Dr. Jorge Plutzky, director of the vascular disease prevention program at Harvard-affiliated Brigham and Women's Hospital, agrees. "The advanced lipoprotein profile is something that the majority of people really don't need." He went on to say, "The reason: there aren't any therapies based on the information the new tests deliver."[67]

In this same article, he did say the people who would benefit from advanced lipid testing might be "a sibling or parent with cardiovascular disease, but no apparent risk factors, or a patient with cardiovascular disease that continues to progress despite aggressive treatment."

---

[67] "'Advanced' cholesterol testing: Is it for you?" https://www.health.harvard.edu/diseases-and-conditions/advanced-cholesterol-testing-is-it-for-you.

LDL particle size is significant. In the literature, small, dense LDL is the most atherogenic. Very low-density lipoprotein (VLDL) can become large, "fluffy" LDL or small, dense LDL. The smaller LDL is more easily oxidized and penetrates the endothelium almost two times more than the large, buoyant LDL. HDL cholesterol can be HDL2 or HDL3, and the HDL2 is better.

Apolipoprotein B resides on every VLDL, LDL, and intermediate-density lipoprotein (IDL) and is a marker for the amount of these lipoproteins. An elevation in this marker can increase your patient's risk of heart disease nearly two and a half times.

"There is considerable evidence that concentrations of Apo B and LDL-particle concentration … are superior indicators of vascular/heart disease driving physiology than either total cholesterol or LDL-cholesterol."[68]

Myleoperoxidase (MPO), often reported on the advanced lipid panel, is a marker of inflammation, frequently found in unstable plaque. Along the lines of inflammatory markers more specific to vascular health, you might include hs-CRP and LP-PLA2. High levels of HsCRP correlate directly with endothelial permeability, whereas LPPLA2 is reported as a direct indicator of vascular inflammation. A 2008 article in *American Journal of Cardiology* announced "Lp-PLA2 determination may provide a pivotal opportunity to appropriately classify previously misclassified persons who are actually at high risk of stroke and in need of aggressive stroke intervention."[69]

---

[68] A. Sachdeva, C. P. Cannon, P. C. Deedwania, et al., "For the Get with the Guidelines Steering Committee and Hospitals. Lipid levels in patients hospitalized with coronary artery disease: an analysis of 136,905 hospitalizations in Get with the Guidelines," *Am Heart J* 157(1)(2009): 111–117.e2.

[69] Gorelick, "Lipoprotein-associated phospholipase A2 and risk of stroke," *Am J Cardiol* 101(12A)(2008): 34F–40F, DOI: 10.1016/j.amjcard.2008.04.017.

TIP

Excellent comprehensive guidelines for cholesterol, from AHA/ACC/AACVPR/AAPA/ABC/ACPM/ADA/AGS/APhA/ASPC/NLA/PCNA can be found at https://www.ahajournals.org/doi/10.1161/CIR.0000000000000625.

TIP

Carotid intima-medial thickness (CIMT) and calcium coronary scanning have demonstrated promising results for early detection of heart disease and prevention for stroke. CIMT testing measures the thickness of the inner two layers of the carotid: the intima and the media. It is a simple ultrasound scan that can alert physicians and patients to potential asymptomatic early disease.

I find this tool to be useful in the office. Most of my patients appreciate tangible evidence as we follow their lifestyle modifications.

Fast Fact

50 percent of heart attacks leading to sudden death happen in patients with normal cholesterol.[70]

Clearly, optimal blood pressure and cholesterol regulation would be beneficial to your patients, but hopefully it is obvious we can also help reduce health-care costs even if this is the only area you apply function

---

[70] Leticia Fernández-Friera, MD, PhD, Valentín Fuster, MD, PhD, Beatriz López-Melgar, MD, PhD, Belén Oliva, José M. García-Ruiz, MD, José Mendiguren, MD, Héctor Bueno, MD, PhD, Stuart Pocock, MSC, PhD, Borja Ibáñez, MD, PhD, Antonio Fernández-Ortiz, MD, PhD, Javier Sanz, MD, "Normal LDL-Cholesterol Levels Are Associated with Subclinical Atherosclerosis in the Absence of Risk Factors," *Journal of the American College Of Cardiology* 70(24)(2017), https://doi.org/10.1016/j.jacc.2017.10.024.

primary care. It is my hope you think of the pathology presenting, and with simple application of the above-mentioned recommendations, I foresee a happier day-to-day practice and healthier patient population.

ADDITIONAL RESOURCES FOR HYPERTENSION AND CHOLESTEROL

1. Gorelick, "Lipoprotein-associated phospholipase A2 and risk of stroke," *Am J Cardiol* 101(12A)(2008): 34F–40F, DOI: 10.1016/j.amjcard.2008.04.017.
2. J. S. Lim, D. H. Lee, J. Y. Park, S. H. Jin, and D. R. Jacobs, "Reliability of low-density lipoprotein cholesterol, non-high-density lipoprotein cholesterol, and apolipoprotein B measurement," *Journal of Clinical Lipidology* 5(4)(2011): 264.
3. T. A. Jacobson, "Opening a new lipid 'apothecary': incorporating apolipoproteins as potential risk factors and treatment targets to reduce cardiovascular risk," *Mayo Clinic Proceedings* 86(8) (2011): 762–780, DOI:10.4065/mcp.2011.0128, PMC 3146376, PMID 21803958.
4. *The Lancet* 344(8934)(1994): 1383–1389.
5. "Prevention of Cardiovascular Events and Death with Pravastatin in Patients with Coronary Heart Disease and a Broad Range of Initial Cholesterol Levels," *N Engl J Med* 339(1998): 1349–1357.
6. The Long-Term Intervention with Pravastatin in Ischemic Disease (LIPID) Study Group.
7. CDC Foundation, "Heart Disease and Stroke Cost America Nearly $1 Billion A Day In Medical Costs, Lost Productivity" (April 29, 2015).
8. "Levels of Evidence Supporting American College of Cardiology/American Heart Association and European Society of Cardiology Guidelines, 2008–2018."
9. Leticia Fernández-Friera, MD, PhD, Valentín Fuster, MD, PhD, Beatriz López-Melgar, MD, PhD, Belén Oliva, José M. García-Ruiz, MD, José Mendiguren, MD, Héctor Bueno, MD, PhD, Stuart Pocock, MSC, PhD, Borja Ibáñez, MD,

PhD, Antonio Fernández-Ortiz, MD, PhD, Javier Sanz, MD, "Normal LDL-Cholesterol Levels Are Associated With Subclinical Atherosclerosis in the Absence of Risk Factors," *Journal of the American College Of Cardiology* 70(24)(2017), https://doi.org/10.1016/j.jacc.2017.10.024.

CHAPTER EIGHT

DIABETES/INSULIN RESISTANCE

As functional PCPs in the making, it seems more prudent to discuss pre-diabetes. Maybe it's even better if we think pre-pre-diabetes, also known as insulin resistance, a topic that truly could have a book of its own. I have no doubt understanding the pathogenesis of insulin resistance and subsequent sequela will change the way you approach your patients. Insulin resistance contributes to comorbidities including, but unfortunately not limited to, cardiovascular, bone, and liver health, all of which are reversible when functional medicine physicians practice true preventive medicine.

Diabetes and insulin resistance are increasing at an astronomical rate and is now spanning across almost all ages.

> The American Diabetes Association suggests a HgbA1C less than 7.0 percent for non-pregnant adults, which equates to an average blood glucose greater than 154.

I feel the ultimate goal should always be prevention; thus waiting until my patients present with a HgbA1C of 7.0 percent seems poor practice. I understand it takes education from the clinician to the patient, and if you do not have the time, there are many ways to tackle this obstacle. Group visits are an excellent solution. Whatever your resolution to this need for extra education, which will result in more patient compliance, I suggest you start early and keep the hgbA1C less than 5.6 percent.

The most impactful bit of data in the literature I share with my patients is the fact that now we know neurologist refer to dementia as type 3 diabetes and approximately every year your HgA1c is above 5.6 percent your average brain volume loss is 1 percent.[71]

PATHOGENESIS SIMPLIFIED

With high amounts of blood glucose, cells become resistant to insulin transport, the body deposits more fat cells to compensate, and more fat cells (besides getting a bigger waist) increase inflammation. Inflammatory cascade is elicited all over, including intravascular. There is an increase in oxidized LDL, causing more endothelial damage, calcification, and plaque progression, thus leading to hardening of the arteries, less compliance/elasticity, and less blood flow to the brain and increase in cardiovascular diseases such as hypertension (and, of course, hypercholesterolemia).

Ideally, I prefer to catch the progression before the HgA1c is greater than 5.4 percent.

Fast Fact

Microvascular damage starts approximately ten years before the diagnosis of diabetes.[72]

---

[71] C. Enzinger¹, F. Fazekas, P. M. Matthews, S. Ropele, H. Schmidt, S. Smith, and R. Schmidt, "Risk factors for progression of brain atrophy in aging: six-year follow-up of normal subjects," Neurology 64(10)(2005): 1704–1711.

[72] D. S. Fong, L. P. Aiello, F. L. Ferris 3rd, and R. Klein, "Diabetic retinopathy," *Diabetes Care* 27(2004): 2540–2553, PMID: 15451934, DOI: 10.2337/diacare.27.10.2540.

I do this by further investigation. I order a fasting insulin and postprandial glucose level or glucose tolerance test, if the HgA1C is between 5.5 and 6.4 percent.[73],[74]

Fast Fact

Insulin resistance contributes to osteoporosis too!

Cellular resistance to sustained hyperglycemia leads to brittle bones ... by way of decreasing osteoblasts, thus increasing osteoclast.

Another alarming, yet interesting, physiologic relationship is found between hyperglycemia and fatty liver disease. Increased blood glucose increases serum-free fatty acids, triglycerides, and inflammatory markers, which lead to hepatocyte damage and fibrosis.

Pre-diabetes (insulin resistance) treatment obviously consists of diet and lifestyle support, but also remember that metformin is a great second-line treatment but can deplete B12. Replacement may be needed.

I use several macronutrients as well. NAC, Berberine, chromium picolinate, COQ10, magnesium, vitamin D, and alpha lipoic acid are especially important with enough literature to support their use. Replacing nutrients and prescribing medicine are all secondary prevention, so let us not forget the simple tape measure is an indispensable primary prevention tool. Performing a waist-to-hip ratio (WHR) as part of your patient's vitals takes little time, and this metric is truly a good return on investment. In the *JAMA* suggested literature, men with WHR greater than 0.90 and females with WHR greater than 0.08 are

---

[73] Optimal goal range less than 3–5 uIU/mL has better outcomes, but current recommendations suggest less than 8.

[74] J. L. Johnson, D. S. Duick, M. A. Chui, and S. A. Aldasouqi, "Identifying prediabetes using fasting insulin levels," *Endocr Pract* 16(1)(2010): 47–52, DOI: 10.4158/EP09031.

at moderate increase risk for poor health, especially cardiovascular and diabetes. Some argue a WHR below 0.5 is best![75]

Metformin depletes B12. B12 deficiency presents with neuropathic pain often. Diabetics usually develop neuropathy in the course of diagnosis. It's awful if the medicine we are giving them is contributing to this. The mechanism of action is related to calcium antagonism. You do not have to stop the medicine. Just replace the nutrients (calcium and B12) if needed.

For example, a publication in 2016 *Gynecological Endocrinology Journal* mentioned the positive effects of N-acetyl cysteine 600 milligrams three times daily in pre-diabetic women/PCOS. It has better efficacy than 500 milligrams metformin (equal frequency) in lowering triglycerides and fasting glucose and insulin.[76]

Being aware of the potential pharmacological-induced deficiency is an excellent way to support your patient's need of these effective medications. Relative to insulin resistance and cardiovascular disease, melatonin and COQ10 are decreased with beta-blocking agents, and sulfonylureas can lower CoQ10. Angiotensin inhibitors are important in the preservation of renal function and cardiac remodeling; nonetheless, it is wise to replace deficiencies of zinc, if necessary.

I recommend you follow nutrient levels the best you can. Testing is available, specifically serum, urine, and hair, and the good ol' physical exam. Be familiar and comfortable with them and follow results to guide your treatment.

---

[75] Connor A. Emdin, DPhil, Amit V. Khera, MD, Pradeep Natarajan, MD, et al., "Genetic Association of Waist-to-Hip Ratio With Cardiometabolic Traits, Type 2 Diabetes, and Coronary Heart Disease," *JAMA* (February 14, 2017), DOI:10.1001/jama.2016.21042.

[76] F. Javanmanesh, M. Kashanian, M. Rahimi, and N. Sheikhansari "A comparison between the effects of metformin and N-acetyl cysteine (NAC) on some metabolic and endocrine characteristics of women with polycystic ovary syndrome," *Gynecol Endocrinol* 32(4)(2016): 285–289, DOI: 10.3109/09513590.2015.1115974.

If there is one area of potential optimization and prevention that can have profound benefits, it is in the realm of insulin and blood glucose regulation. As primary care clinicians, we can assist our patients in proactive health participation. No one ever says, "I'd rather think slower and be in pain always!" Start now. Change your approach. Implement action before the labs are drastically abnormal and remember the ol' adage "it's in my genes, so I will get it …" is a farce.

ADDITIONAL RESOURCES FOR DIABETES

1. J. L. Johnson, D. S. Duick, M. A. Chui, and S. A. Aldasouqi, *World J Diabetes* 2(3)(2011): 41–48, DOI:0.4239/wjd.v2.i3.41.
2. Kannikar Wongdee and Narattaphol Charoenphandhu, "Osteoporosis in diabetes mellitus: Possible cellular and molecular mechanisms," PMCID: PMC3083906, PMID: 21537459.
3. Y. Kumeda, "Osteoporosis in diabetes," *Clin Calcium* 18(5) (2008): 589–599, DOI: CliCa0805589599.
4. *International Journal of Endocrinology* (2014), http://dx.doi.org/10.1155/2014/820615.
5. Peter Jackuliak and Juraj Payer, "Osteoporosis, Fractures, and Diabetes."
6. E. Bugianesi, S. Moscatiello, M. F. Ciaravella, and G. Marchesini, "Insulin resistance in nonalcoholic fatty liver disease," *Curr Pharm Des* 16(17)(2010): 1941–1951.
7. Hironori Kitade, Guanliang Chen, Yinhua Ni, and Tsuguhito Ota, "Nonalcoholic Fatty Liver Disease and Insulin Resistance: New Insights and Potential New Treatments," *Nutrients* 9(4) (2017): 387, DOI: 10.3390/nu9040387, PMCID: PMC5409726, PMID: 28420094.

CHAPTER NINE

GENETICS

I have referred to genetic testing throughout the book, and I will give a very brief overview of a few common nutrigenomic single nucleotide polymorphisms (SNPs) and medical genomics that I find useful in primary care. Genetics are not our end-all-be-all.[77]

For me, identifying the GSTP1 variant was monumental in my health recovery. When I started glutathione replacement with high-dose replacement (750 milligrams per day), I reduced the ulcerations in my oral mucosa by 50 percent in less than two days. This was not a one-time occurrence, but it is my go-to if I feel a flare on the horizon. It works without a doubt.

Fast Fact

GSTP1 is involved in over two hundred different diseases, including a variety of cancers due to the important role GSTP1 plays in detoxifying carcinogens and "G" allele is associated with, elevated mercury levels.

---

[77] Johns Hopkins Medical Institutions, "Our Genome Changes Over Lifetime, And May Explain Many 'Late-onset' Diseases," ScienceDaily, June 25, 2008.

Individualization of medicine is where we are headed! With companies such as 23andMe, Mayo Clinic's GeneGuide, GENESIGHT, Genomind (for psychiatric pharmacokenetics), and, my favorite, IntellXXDNA, identifying your patient's genomics is inexpensive and readily available. The results, in my opinion, should be used as a guide for your clinical decisions, not as a diagnostic tool. I do recommend you not order these tests if you are not able to fully study the details and feel confident to review the results with your patients. It is an ever-evolving field of science, so choose wisely.

For the PCP, if you feel like you want to keep it simple, there are a few that particularly pertain to cardiovascular health that can be ordered as a standard blood draw. MTHFR, APO B/Apo A1, and APO E3 and APOE 4 are a few of my favorites. All have substantial publications and research to support their usefulness in preventive cardiometabolic health.

Let me help with straightforward definitions and how I apply the information in clinical practice.

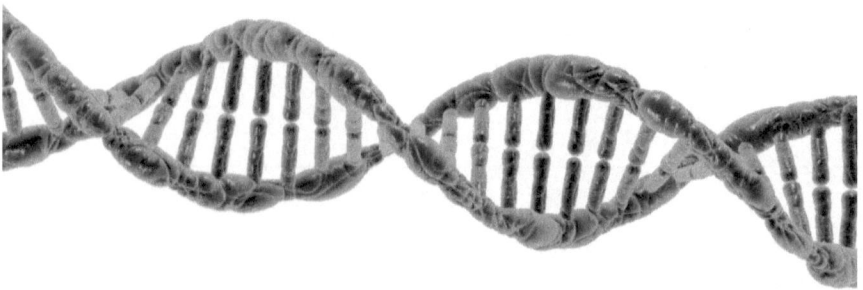

DNA

First, a little basic genetic review:

Chromosomes are the most macro view of our genes; inside the chromosome are our genes, twenty-three pairs (one part from mom and one part from dad). These genes are made up of amino acids ATCG that combine in many patterns to make a protein, which make up exons and introns. Most of our DNA are introns, and we only know little of what they do! It is a dynamic and ever-expanding field of research!

Your lab report will likely list results in this basic format: normal, +- heterozygote, ++ homozygous.

Heterozygosity means one allele normal and one allele abnormal. (This never tells us whether it is mutated to be upregulated or downregulated.) Homozygous mutations mean both alleles are abnormal. Single nucleotide polymorphisms appear when a nucleotide (building block) of the genome is changed for another nucleotide. Most of the SNPs—and there are many—have no known health implications (though I am humbled by the amount of new information I feel almost on a minute-to-minute basis).

When one nucleotide is swapped for another, however, it can alter the function of that particular enzyme. The life-altering SNPs are detected early in life; however, there are many that alter a pathway or the person's biochemistry subtly. This subtle alteration in function can result in increased health risks or even suboptimal function.

Methyl-tetrahydrofolate reductase is one heck of a Scrabble word! MTHFR, for short, is an enzyme responsible for many processes, but for the sake of this section, I will focus on cardiovascular implications if this is defective. Specifically, this enzyme converts 5, 10 methylene-tetrahydrafolate to the simplified 5 methyltetrahydrofolate, and this is important for the conversion of homocysteine to methionine. High levels of homocysteine can increase a person's risk of endothelial damage. Vessel wall damage can, of course, increase inflammatory reactions, thus leading to atherogenesis. Hyper-homocysteinemia, even mild, has been associated with increased risk of stroke and ischemic cardiovascular and poorer post-stroke events.[78] It also has been associated with increase in neural tube defects.

---

[78] Min Zhao, X. Wang, M. He, X. Qin, G. Tang, et al., "Homocystiene and Stroke—Modifying effect of MTHFR C677T polymorphism and folic acid intervention," *Stroke* 48(2017): 1183–1190.

Therefore, if you see a homocysteine higher than 8–10 micromoles/L (most labs rr is 4-15), it is contributing to ROS and inflammation, specifically known to affect the vascular system. Start addressing it here. I recommend you do not wait for your patient's homocysteine to increase to 12–14 before implementing lifestyle modifications (a diet high in leafy and dark greens and adding in bioavailable B12/folate).

The reason for a bioavailable supplementation, in the case of MTHFR SNPs, is the poor ability to methylate. Thus, adding vitamin B9 and B12 in the methylated form will help with this process. As an additional tip, adding trimethylglycine has also shown to help because, in the liver, Betaine-Homocysteine S-Methyltransferase (BHMT) catalyzes up to 50 percent of homocysteine metabolism.[79] I would like to add that this is a small part of the methylation cycle, so be knowledgeable about the pathways, and remember, nothing is one size fits all.

Fast Fact

Shellfish, spinach, and beets are good food sources of betaine.

Slightly related, but lesser known, is that of MTRR C524T and A66G, Methothionine Synthatase. MTRR is necessary to recycle homocysteine, especially in the brain. Activity here is increased by a low methionine level and should be considered as a possible cause of an elevated MCV value. Overall, reduce inflammation and support folate intake.

Lastly, but still related to cardiovascular disease—though documented in fewer studies—is the COMT polymorphisms. COMT val/val and met/met are relative based on Hall et al.'s research, published in 2014 in *Arteriosclerosis, Thrombosis, and Vascular*, titled "Polymorphisms in

---

[79] H. Refsum, P. Ueland, O. Nygard, and S. E. Vollset, "Homocystiene and cardiovascular disease," *Annu Rev Med* 49(1998): 31–62, PMID:9509248, DOI:10.1146.
H. Kwon et al., "Homocystiene as a predictor of early Neurological deterioration in acute ischemic stroke," *Stroke* 45: 871–873, DOI:10.1161.

Catechol-O-methyltransferase Modify Treatment Effects of Aspirin on Risk of Cardiovascular Disease." Essentially, consider aspirin and maybe even vitamin E in Met/Met (mixed tocopherols, in my opinion), and from a CVD prevention standpoint, adding aspirin proves negative in Val/Val.

> **Fast Fact**
>
> Mixed tocopherols is the only vitamin E I recommend, as alpha tocopherol is easily oxidized when alone and dL-alpha tocopherol is the less bioavailable form of vitamin E. Alpha, beta, delta, and gamma tocopherol is how we find vitamin E in nature. Annetto E (delta and gamma tocotrienols) has promising studies for plaque reversal.

APO E 3/3 is the most common genetic makeup that does best with a moderate fat diet, and this population type responds favorably to fish oil supplementation. APO E4/4 and APO E3/4 does best with a low-fat diet. Low simple carbs (especially alcohol) and fish oil helps lower small, dense LDL but raises total LDL. (Be careful advising patients if your information is based solely on the standard lipid panel.)

> **Fast Fact**
>
> APOE4 increases Alzheimer's by 10 to 15 percent if combined with high-fat and high-glycemic diet and induces insulin resistance in the brain (reported by *Neuroscientists in Neuron* in 2017, "Type 3 diabetes"[80]).

Just when we thought we had it all figured out, for the thyroid, it gets more interesting. For practitioners evaluating, diagnosing, and treating a patient with a thyroid disorder, there must be consideration given to the role genetics play. Especially if we are to be comprehensive, we

---

[80] Zhao et al., "Apolipoprotein E4 Impairs Neuronal Insulin Signaling by Trapping Insulin Receptor in the Endosomes," *Neuron* 96(2017): 115–129.

must know not only does stress/perceived stress/HPA function affect optimal thyroid function, but so do genetics, particularly in conversion. "Polymorphism Thr92Ala in *DIO2* is related to lower serum FT3 levels after thyroidectomy, and the D2-Ala mutant reduces T4 to T3 conversion in cell cultures."[81]

As you can see, with the basic genetic variant testing available, one can tailor their patient's treatment accordingly. Personalized medicine is, in my opinion, where medicine is headed. Start with one or two, and with this small implementation, you can improve patient outcomes and satisfaction!

ADDITIONAL RESOURCES FOR GENETICS

1. Q. Feng, K. Kalari, B. L. Fridley, G. Jenkins, Y. Ji, and R. Abo, "Betaine-homocysteine methyltransferase: human liver genotype-phenotype correlation," *Mol Genet Metab* 102(2) (2011): 126–133.
2. *Gynecol Endocrinol* 32(4)(2016): 285–289, DOI: 10.3109/09513590.2015.1115974.
3. F. Javanmanesh, M. Kashanian, M. Rahimi, and N. Sheikhansari, "A comparison between the effects of metformin and N-acetyl cysteine (NAC) on some metabolic and endocrine characteristics of women with polycystic ovary syndrome," *Gynecol Endocrinol* 32(4)(2016): 285–289, DOI: 10.3109/09513590.2015.1115974.
4. L. F. Masson, G. McNeill, and A. Avenell, "Genetic variation and the lipid response to dietary intervention: a systematic review," *Am J Clin Nutr* 77(5)(2003): 1098–111.
5. D. Corella, K. Tucker, C. Lahoz, O. Coltell, L. A. Cupples, P. W. Wilson, E. J. Schaefer, and J. M. Ordovas, "Alcohol drinking determines the effect of the APOE locus on LDL-cholesterol

---

[81] Wilmar M Wiersinga, "Therapy of Endocrine Disease T4+T3 combination therapy: is there a true effect?" *European Journal of Endocrinology* 177(6)(2017): R287–R296.

concentrations in men: the Framingham Offspring Study," *Am J Clin Nutr* 73(4)(2001): 736–745.
6. Y. Song, M. J. Stampfer, and S. Liu, "Meta-analysis: Apolipoprotein E genotypes and risk for coronary heart disease," *Ann Intern Med* 141(2004): 137–147.
7. J. Lopez-Miranda et al., "Effect of apolipoprotein E phenotype on diet-induced lowering of plasma low density lipoprotein cholesterol," *J Lipid Res* 35(1994): 1965–1975.
8. J. Moreno et al., "The effect of dietary fat on LDL size is influenced by apolipoprotein E genotype in healthy subjects," *J Nutr* 134(2004): 2517–2522.11.
9. D. J. Jenkins, R. A. Hegele, A. L. Jenkins, P. W. Connelly, K. Hallak, P. Bracci, and R. Bruce, "The apolipoprotein E gene and the serum low-density lipoprotein cholesterol response to dietary fiber," *Metabolism* 42(5)(1993): 585–593.
10. Kwon et al. (2014), Petras et al. (2014), Williams et al. (2014), Refusm et al. (1998).
11. H. Refsum, P. Ueland, O. Nygard, and S. E. Vollset, "Homocystiene and cardiovascular disease," Annu Rev Med 49(1998): 31–62.
12. H. Kwon et al., "Homocystiene as a predictor of early Neurological deterioration in cute ischemic stroke," *Stroke* 45: 871–873.
13. Min Zhao et al., "Homocystiene and Stroke—Modifying effect of MTHFR C677T polymorphism and folic acid intervention," *Stroke* 48(2017): 1183–1190.
14. Genetics play a large role in hypercholesterolemia. Research suggests 93 percent of patients with LDL greater than 190 likely has a genetic SNP LDLR family member with one or the other, total LDL greater than 190, or premature heart disease.
15. IntellXX DNA report
16. V. Andreoli et al., "Genetic Aspects of Susceptibility to Mercury Toxicity: An Overview," *Int J Environ Res Public Health* 14(1) (2017): 93.

CHAPTER TEN

LAB ORDERS: WHAT WILL BE YOUR BIGGEST RETURN ON INVESTMENT (ROI)?

WHAT LABS SHOULD YOU CONSIDER?

I suggest you research your local sources and ask what they have available. You may be surprised to learn they carry several preventive panels. Quest or LabCorp have comprehensive cholesterol panels and homocysteine. Most labs I use require a blood draw or urine samples. You should start with the basics, in the name of cost (both to the patient and the insurance company) and add only if and when necessary. For example, if their homocysteine is elevated, then I recommend MMA and serum B12, folate, and MTHFR, but I do not start with all of those.

From my experience, both Quest and LabCorp have advanced cholesterol panels. The more you familiarize yourself with advanced lipid testing, the more you may decide to add this to your preventive panel. The other labs on my requisition speak for themselves. TSH and free T3/T4, vit D 25 OH, CMP, CBC, fasting insulin, glucose tolerance test, serum glutathione (optional), and CoQ10 levels (optional).

A favorite specialty test of mine is one to assess overall nutrient status. (Yes, this fluctuates moment to moment, but it is a nice way to get an overall picture of your patient's nutrient status.) There are several comprehensive nutrient panels. The one we used at Cleveland Clinic Center for Functional Medicine is the one with which I am most familiar, Nutra Eval by Genova Diagnostics. This is a serum and urine metabolic nutrient assessment of vitamins (metabolites), minerals, amino acids, omega 3-6-9-7, and antioxidants.

A second specialty test I often use in my practice is a comprehensive stool test. This is for many primary care patients who present with IBS and gastrointestinal complaints. The structural investigation most often proves to be normal. Esophagogastroduodenoscopy (EGD) and colonoscopy reveal no etiology for their complaints. This is why microscopic testing is beneficial. PCR and culture tests prove to be helpful in many cases. Commensal microbiome balance is key for proper immune, hormonal, and neurotransmitter function. A culture of three to four weeks can be additionally helpful to identify potential pathogenic bacteria and even more successful when accompanied with a treatment sensitivity panel. There are several comprehensive stool tests on the market. I appreciate the comprehensive information from a Clinical Laboratory Improvement Amendments (CLIA)-certified lab. I utilize the information of B-glucuronidase levels, short-chain fatty acid levels, mycology and parasitic cultures, and microscopic analysis, to mention a few.

Last, but not least, educate yourself! Continuing medical education (CME) is important, and as rapidly as information is printed, it is difficult to stay on top of the research. I feel this is a great time to mention the cardiometabolic advance module offered by the Institute for Functional Medicine (IFM), an excellent CME. If you appreciate the information in this book, you will not be disappointed. IFM conferences are highly recommended. (No, I do not have stock or vested interest in the company.)

CHAPTER ELEVEN

CASE EXAMPLE: FUNCTIONAL PRIMARY CARE

CASE EXAMPLE

Mr. X presents to the office with complaint of uncontrolled hypertension and heart racing. This patient is a fifty-year-old male who thinks he has had high blood pressure on and off for a few years but noticed it really has been a problem every time he has it checked this last year. His work offered a physical at a health screening, and they suggested he see his doctor.

He reluctantly gives you a timeline with nothing on it—healthy as a child, healthy as an adult, and healthy now. After pressing further, he admits he is caffeine dependent, with four cups or more per day, because he "can't get going or stay going without it." He admits also about three years ago he started having more restless nights of sleep and has been having some headaches, especially after a stressful day.

As he opens up more, he reports he has noticed more irritability and less excitement or motivation for life in general, though, as do most depressed patients, he denies depression. He still finds pleasure in daily activities. He's just not as motivated. His wife says he's cranky all the time. He still works out in the morning, but he finds that he's not gaining any muscle mass. He feels like he's losing muscle, and he's gaining weight. His heart starts racing, usually in the evening, especially when he lays down to go to bed. His libido is "okay." He denies any erectile dysfunction, although he admits "it doesn't last as long." He also has noticed that his hair loss has increased rapidly over the last year.

Mind you, he is very reluctant to divulge this information. I find it's very difficult for many patients, particularly men and very type-A personalities, to share private information or symptoms that might be perceived as weaknesses. As a physician, I recommend a very gentle approach.

I explain my reasoning for the prying. For example, in this situation, I would explain, "Oftentimes when the thyroid is functioning abnormally or you have a decrease in testosterone, this can affect your cardiovascular system. It is important for me to ask the questions, and I appreciate your honest answers. It helps me provide the best care possible." Once I explained this, Mr. X more readily shares information.

In this case, I ordered some lab work consisting of TSH, free T4, total testosterone, free testosterone, sex-binding globulin hormone, RBC magnesium, potassium, CMP, CBC, CRPHS, nutritional panel, and serum lead. (This will check acute levels, not total body burden.) For Mr. X, I recommend he have a carotid intimal thickening test (CIMT) and variable heart rate (VHR) measurement taken before the next visit.

Variable heart rate is a way of measuring the fluctuations between heart beats. Healthy individuals demonstrate good variability, and unhealthy individual results show poor reactive variability. It is a quick and easy measure of the adaptably of the cardiovascular system as it relates to the sympathetic and parasympathetic nervous system.

Structural assessment is just as feasible in an office visit. CIMT and arterial elasticity can be an early detection for atherosclerosis and vessel resistance according to the American Heart Association 2000 published guidelines. This is a simple noninvasive tool for the office with ample published literature in respected journals such as *Stroke*, *Circulation*, and the *Annals of Internal Medicine*, to name a few.

See the fun fact below for the reason I check lead, especially with cardiovascular complaints.

Fun Fact

Lead was banned in house paint in 1978 and in gasoline in 1985, but it was not completely out until 1995. From the 1950s to 1978, paint had lead in it, and even if you were not using it to paint your house anymore, if you lived in a home painted in that time, you had exposure. It's commonly found in the flaking paint chips or in the soil around the house. Patients who were born in this era have the high potential of lead body burden, especially post-menopause or man-o-pause, because of the increase in bone turnover/loss. Lead can contribute to cardiovascular disease, especially hypertension. Therefore, because my patient was born in 1969, I have lead on my differential. It's not my part of my initial evaluation, but it should be on the list to investigate, if not better, with the basics. Also I feel it best to first optimize the body's own ability for elimination, so it can best excrete toxins like lead. I suggest never implementing patient chelation without proper nutritional, genetic, and biochemical support.

INITIAL RECOMMENDATIONS

- Begin to wean coffee. The goal is two cups per day, max.
- Perform deep breathing once per day, ten to fifteen minutes. I recommended he download a guided mediation/mindfulness. (I felt this was the best place for him to start.) As for dietary

changes, I suggest a green vegetable with all three meals and no white foods (sugar, flour, rice, and potatoes).
- Continue with his workouts, as tolerated.

Four weeks later (a typical ideal follow-up time for my practice), Mr. X should return for his follow-up visit. It will be a follow-up of fifteen minutes, and the focus will be on lab review and a new plan. (Take more time if you have it available.)

Before I get to this patient's follow-up, I have a few points to make relative to this case. In this case example, as with many real patients, I address several abnormalities revealed by the lab tests. I always address the thyroid, known as the master gland. If it is functioning normally, then I say that. If not, then it is the first system I address. (I said "system" because it ties into the adrenals, gonads, pituitary, and hypothalamus.)

> **Tip**
>
> End the last visit with, "At your next visit, we will be pressed for time considering the amount of information I will have gained, so I will be very to the point. I will not rush you, but in order for you to get maximum benefits and a new plan, we will stay focused. Okay?" This sets the tone for the follow-up. Follow-up visits require only pertinent positive and negative lab review, a short bit of time to assess their clinical status and do your physical exam. (I usually inquire about their last four weeks while I am examining the patient, and I found the patient can enter in their subjective information, to which you read and add information as needed.)

FOLLOW-UP #1

For the sake of example, this gentleman's TSH is 5.76 and free t4 if 0.6. Free t3 and rT3 were not checked, but I will send him to have these checked before his next visit because of his initial thyroid panel results.

My hope is always, once we give the body what it needs for thyroid conversion, it will improve.

In my experience, this happens often in my practice about 40 percent of the time. Replacing t4 and adding nutrients needed for thyroid T4 to T3 conversion is imperative. And for this patient, this included selenium, zinc, and vitamin D3. (See below for results as all these help in thyroid function). I will include Free t3 (rT3 if he is still tired) in my follow-up lab check in six weeks.

Nonetheless, this is frank hypothyroidism, which could be contributing to his hormone imbalance and heart palpitations. Both his free and total testosterone were low normal. (This is age dependent, mind you.) And his sex hormone binding globulin (SHBG) was high. When the protein-binding globulin level is elevated, it does exactly that: bind sex hormones; therefore, the available "free testosterone" is typically lower.

Tip

One of the best ways to lower the SHBG is to decrease inflammation by cutting out dietary intake of junk food.

Tip

Magnesium citrate can cause loose bowel movements; unless the patient tends toward constipation, I typically use other forms of magnesium, for instance, glycinate, malate, and so forth.

Fast Fact

Magnesium threonate is the only magnesium known to cross the blood-brain barrier.

In this case, because he is a male able to perform activities of daily living, I suggest he first start with thyroid hormone balance and lifestyle modification and then retest testosterone levels. It is worth mentioning, if he were bedridden or debilitated, I would replace testosterone while I did all the above, retesting and decreasing or stopping when not needed. Sometimes it can be a real boost, but like everything we give that alters biochemistry, there are side effects or adverse reaction potentials. I am going to say it again: less is always best when it comes to pharmaceuticals and nutraceuticals. (Hormones fall into these categories.)

His RBC magnesium, RBC zinc, and selenium were low, as was his potassium low normal. The nutritional evaluation panel suggested deficiencies in B6, B3. I recommended a B complex. (I only use a bioavailable B complex because many of the population are poor metabolizers of several B vitamins, i.e., MTHFR, etc.) I added magnesium and zinc replacement. As for the selenium, he was able to get that replacement in his diet.

Fast Fact

With selenium-rich foods, be careful replacing selenium with large non-food doses. Selenium can be toxic.

Shitake mushrooms: 36 micrograms per cooked cup

Brazil nuts (1 handful): 544 micrograms per 28 grams (an adult handful)

Pay close attention to the units of measurement in supplements. Selenium is reported in micrograms, and 800 micrograms daily can potentially cause toxicity. A dose of 5 milligrams is considered lethal for most people.

FOLLOW-UP #2

I saw him eight weeks later. He had labs drawn at six weeks (TSH, free T4/free T3, vitamin D3, total testosterone, and SHBG).

His testosterone levels improved with decreased SHBG and thyroid improvement since his initial visit, so there was no need to replace testosterone in this patient. His heart palpitations ceased as well. I assured him decreasing his caffeine, regulating his thyroid, and lowering his overall stress response with deep breathing had certainly helped everything, including his heart rhythm abnormalities. TSH was improving, and I continued to monitor it every three months until he clinically felt best, with a TSH level goal of less than 2.0. His blood pressure had reduced both systolic and diastolic, and his variable heart rate test also improved. We continued to follow him every three months for two more visits then twice per year. I am happy to report, several years later, he is compliant with his lifestyle and diet and feeling well.

Fun Fact

Magnesium deficiency is not easy to detect, and subclinical deficiency is thought to be rampant, with greater than 80 percent of the population having a deficiency state. Subclinical deficiency of magnesium affects ionic influx/efflux, ATP production and activation, DNA/RNA protein synthesis, and cell structural integrity and plays a role in over three hundred enzymatic processes. Serum magnesium is not a reflection of intracellular magnesium.

Literature review suggests 99 percent of magnesium deficiencies are not diagnosed. A silent decrease in efficiency of the biochemical pathways leads to the subclinical nature. The current recommendation to prevent frank deficiency is 300–420 milligrams per day (RDA). This is not for optimization of function. Sadly, all over the world, the population is not getting this in their daily intake. For example, in the United States, the average intake for women and men is between 228–323 milligrams per day.[82] Check RBC magnesium for best cellular representation.[83] In this case example, as with many real patients, I address several abnormalities revealed by the lab tests. I always address the thyroid, known as the master gland. If it is functioning normally, then I say that. If not, then it is the first system I address. (I said "system" because it ties into the adrenals, gonads, pituitary, and hypothalamus.)

---

[82] Earl S. Ford and Ali H. Mokdad, "Dietary Magnesium Intake in a National Sample of U.S. Adults," *The Journal of Nutrition* 133(9)(2003): 2879–2882, https://doi.org/10.1093/jn/133.9.2879.

[83] Y. Ismail and A. A. Ismail, "The underestimated problem of using serum magnesium measurements to exclude magnesium deficiency in adults; a health warning is needed for 'normal' results," *Clin Chem Lab Med* 48(3)(2010): 323–327, DOI: 10.1515/CCLM.2010.077.

CHAPTER TWELVE

PEDIATRIC CONCERNS: PANS, PANDAS, AND ASD

Family physicians see many children, and the sooner we identify root causes of illnesses, the better. I would like to point out a couple topics of interest. All the above recommendations can be applied to the pediatric population reference ranges. Adjust for age accordingly.

Let's look at pediatric acute-onset neuropsychiatric syndrome (PANS), pediatric autoimmune neuropsychiatric disorders associated with streptococcal infections (PANDAS), and autism spectrum disorders (ASD). I feel the breadth of knowledge for physicians is limited when it comes to PANS, PANDAS, and ASD, hence the reason for me to add this short section.

This is a personal area of interest. My journey navigating my daughter's health challenges continues to teach me so very much. This is a journey for another book, but I feel for those parents who know something is wrong with their child and cannot get anyone to listen. It is similar to being the patient and being ignored and pushed away or labeled as "crazy." But it's worse because this is your child, a sweet immature human who depends on you to be their advocate. PANS and PANDAS diagnoses are fairly new neuropsychological disorders.

I first heard of PANDAS and sensory integrative disorder (SIDS) in residency in 2008. This was at a continuing medical education lecture by the PANS/PANDAS leading researcher from National Institutes for Mental Health, Dr. Swedo, who presented the newest research suggesting an infectious etiology for some children's OCD, tic, and abnormal behavioral tendencies. At the time, it was a hypothesis, "a potential cause for a sudden change in a child's neuropsychological baseline following a recent infection." Eventually several researchers presented enough evidence to achieve a DSM-IV diagnosis code. Then finally in 2012 and 2017, new NIMH guidelines have since been established and updated (https://www.nimh.nih.gov/health/publications/pandas/index.shtml).

I am not an expert, but there are several physicians—immunologists, neurologists, and psychologists—who do specialize in this disorder. This NIH.gov website is an excellent referral source, as is pandasnetwork.org.

ASDs are increasingly being diagnosed, and early detection continues to be most important for improved outcomes. This disorder is inclusive of sensory processing disorder (SPD), Asperger's, and autism. These are all on the autism spectrum of diagnoses, and patients can have varying degrees of severity. Some are high functioning, and others are challenged with common activities of daily living. I have personal experience with this spectrum and realize earliest interventions are best. Diet and lifestyle, especially in the arena of proper sleep and optimal nutrition replacement, has proven to be very impactful with my ASD patients. Identifying and removing any insults to the inflammatory response in these children also have strong positive improvements.

I know there is an incredible amount of concern around vaccinations as the cause of this disorder. I do not feel vaccinations are the sole cause, but after seeing over a thousand children on the spectrum, I can say the timing is concerning. I feel this diagnosis is just as individual as all the above presentations. It is my educated theory. Several, if not all, systems play a role. Genetics, poor gastrointestinal health, and the resultant poor nutrient status in these patients create increased total body oxidative stress. With all of that brewing, around two years old we add insult to injury and expose this imbalanced system to a large amount of immune stimulation (from vaccinations), and for some, this may be the perfect storm.

For those concerned about giving their children vaccinations, I recommend supporting genetically impaired conjugation pathways and phase 1 biotransformation (detoxification) before and after vaccination administration. (The identification of genetic polymorphisms for neurobehavior dysfunction is in the investigative stages, and I am honored to be part of this group of physicians.) Proper investigation into the basic functional medicine-matrix categories with optimal system restoration has not ever hurt any of my patients, and for some, it has been positively life-altering.

CHAPTER THIRTEEN

TICK-BORNE ILLNESS, INCLUDING LYME DISEASE AND POST-LYME SYNDROME

TICK-BORNE ILLNESS

Reflecting, I am sure, though I admit I cannot be 100 percent certain, I had a tick-borne illness when I was eight to ten years old. I do know I took many herbs that have documented antibacterial and antiparasitic properties, and as I shared, I made improvements in my health after the herbal support protocols were followed.

Also consider Lyme disease, Bartonella, Babesia, anaplasmosis, and so forth. I'm not an expert; however, I must share my disclaimer. I have received basic training by two leading experts in the field, and I am a past member of International Lyme and Associated Diseases Society (ILADS). As controversial as it is, I do believe we are undertreating and underdiagnosing tick illness. Still I am concerned about some of the treatments, especially the one-size-fits-all approach.

Tick illness is real and needs to be treated. The testing we have available is poor and lacking in research.[84] It is nevertheless, per CDC, a clinical diagnosis. The treatment, in my opinion, should be individual and as simple as possible with less amount of biochemical alteration as possible to restore quality of life.

I do feel we need to stop attacking well-meaning physicians for treating patients. This results in fear—fear to discuss tick illness, fear to treat it, and fear to refer.

> Fear is generated from a belief or threat of potential danger, most often based on a lack of knowledge. It is wise to be cautious, but if you let fear stop you from moving forward, you will stop growing.

I feel it is important to share some of my experience. I have treated hundreds of patients whom presented with positive tick bite history, conclusive diagnostic lab results, and symptoms strongly suggestive of tick illness. Migratory joint pain, headaches, occipital neck pain, strange stretch marks, muscle pain, fever, night sweats, and cognitive and mood changes, to name a few common symptoms.

My method of treatment is methodical, although fluctuating. Base the treatment on the patient and their capacity to fight for the restoration of their health. Be flexible and change the modalities and treatment regimen according to their body's response.

Often, once we replaced nutrients, optimized gut health, decreased inflammation, and minimized the stress response, they were able to fight the infection or persistent symptoms of a post infection. The body

---

[84] Institute of Medicine (US) Committee on Lyme Disease and Other Tick-Borne Diseases: The State of the Science. Washington (DC): National Academies Press (US); 2011. Critical Needs and Gaps in Understanding Prevention, Amelioration, and Resolution of Lyme and Other Tick-Borne Diseases: The Short-Term and Long-Term Outcomes: Workshop Report.

is able to restore to homeostasis. I found this to be more common than not. Thus, limiting the amount of chemical treatments is needed.

For example, I will present two patients whom had a CDC criteria diagnosis of Lyme. Both had significant restoration of quality of life, but each one had a different treatment plan.

PATIENT #1

He is a fifty-two-year-old male farmer. He presented being diagnosed with Lyme and Bartonella two months prior to his visit with me. He complained of severe headaches and joint pain that would come and go and "move around." He also had a sudden change in sleep. For two weeks, he was not able to sleep. He had no fever and no night sweats. He received ten days of doxycycline. He had a large bull's-eye rash that was still present and had not received any treatment before presenting to my office.

PATIENT #2

He is a sixty-four-year-old male. He is a hunter. He was diagnosed approximately six weeks before I saw him as a patient. He presented with headaches, neck pain, night sweats, and severe debilitating joint pain. He was active and healthy prior to his tick bites. (He reported his headaches were a lot better while being treated but returned worse after he stopped the doxycycline.)

Patient #1 also had a history of significant constipation. Patient #2 had no prior medical history and denied any other significant history. Nutrient panel for both men revealed a few deficiencies, and I started replacement. For Patient #1, magnesium replacement improved bowel movements, and comprehensive stool test PCR indicated low levels of bifidobacterium, so this too was replaced, and I imagine this helped too.

Patient #1 was given eleven more days of doxycycline, as ten to twenty-one days is the current CDC guideline. He was again headache- and joint pain-free on the antibiotics. I added a few herbal combinations from the Byron White and Zhang formulations for support, and he continued this treatment for two months. After eight weeks, our attempt to wean off the herbal support proved to be challenging as his symptoms returned approximately three days after cessation. We, therefore, continued and adjusted the combinations every three to four weeks until he was symptom free for four months consecutively. Then I weaned him off the treatment. Of note, he continued his nutrition support the entire time. He has remained symptom-free for two years.

Patient #2 was given twenty-one days of doxycycline and *Uncaria tomentosa*,[85] and because of his night sweats, I tested for Babesia by PCR, which was positive, so additionally we started him on Mepron for ten days. This was then followed by an herbal combo that targets protozoans, for which he attempted to stop after four weeks, to no avail. I recommended he continue this herbal combo, and we added a biofilm disruptor, whole leaf stevia from nutramedix,[86] and grapefruit seed extract for potential cyst forms of Borrellia. Eventually we were able to wean him slowly, but after nine months, his symptoms abated. He too continued on nutrition support throughout the entire treatment course.

Here are a few questions I get all the time regarding tick illnesses:

- **Do I believe patients can have reoccurring infection?** Yes.
- **Do I believe patients can have persistent symptoms of tick illness?** Yes. The CDC recognizes a percentage of patients

---

[85] Anna Goc and Matthias Rath, "The anti-borreliae efficacy of phytochemicals and micronutrients: an update," *Ther Adv Infect Dis* 3(3–4)(2016): 75–82, PMCID: PMC4971593, PMID: 27536352, DOI: 10.1177/2049936116655502.

[86] P. Theophilus and M. J. Victoria, "Effectiveness of Stevia Rebaudiana Whole Leaf Extract Against the Various Morphological Forms of Borelia Burgdorferi in Vitro," *European Journal of Microbiology and Immunology* 5(4)(2015): 1–13, DOI: 10.1556/1886.2015.00031.

infected with Borrellia can have chronic post-Lyme symptoms. Symptoms vary but are similar to acute Lyme.
- **Am I certain it is ongoing or a reactivation of the tick infection, as opposed to a triggered immune response with similar presentation?** No.
- **Do I know/believe Borellia illness is only an acute process?** No. The literature most recently presented suggests it is a persistent and immune evasive spirochete.
- **Am I cautious about the use of antibiotics?** Yes. Absolutely!
- **Do I use antibiotics?** Yes, if needed, as in the examples above. If labs and history support the need for antibiotic treatment.

"The Centers for Disease Control and Prevention (CDC) report that at least 300,000 people are infected with Lyme disease each year in the United States."[87]

I recommend a thorough history, and don't forget the testing available is limited.

"In the first three weeks after infection, the test only detects Lyme 29 to 40 percent of the time. (The test is 87 percent accurate once Lyme spreads to the neurological system, and 97 percent accurate for patients who develop Lyme arthritis). The CDC cautions that because the test is not likely to be positive until 4 to 6 weeks after infection, doctors who suspect Lyme based on symptoms should prescribe antibiotics even if the test is negative."[88]

Therefore, if you suspect your patient has a tick-borne illness, treat them with doxycycline or an appropriate alternative for twenty-one days and assess after treatment. And I recommend you optimize the patient's nutrient status.

---

[87] "Data and Surveillance," https://www.cdc.gov/lyme/datasurveillance/index.html.
[88] Catherine Caruso, "Tests for Lyme disease miss many early cases—but a new approach could help," https://www.statnews.com/2017/06/28/early-lyme-tests.

Tick-borne illness is a serious concern and a fast-growing epidemic. As PCPs, if you do not understand the presenting illness, whether it be tick illness, PANS, PANDAS, chronic fatigue, or fibromyalgia, please do your patient a favor and refer them to someone who does know.

ADDITIONAL RESOURCES PANDAS AND TICK-BORNE ILLNESS

Institute of Medicine (US) Committee on Lyme Disease and Other Tick-Borne Diseases: The State of the Science. Washington (DC): National Academies Press (US); 2011. Critical Needs and Gaps in Understanding Prevention, Amelioration, and Resolution of Lyme and Other Tick-Borne Diseases: The Short-Term and Long-Term Outcomes: Workshop Report.

In this chapter of National Academies sponsored by the NIH, "three researchers explored the limitations of existing tests for Lyme borreliosis and other tick-borne diseases and suggested promising new approaches to diagnostics that can improve the diagnosis of those diseases, and four clinicians discussed the challenges and needs for improving diagnosis in the medical office."

https://www.nimh.nih.gov/health/publications/pandas/index.shtml

A NOTE FROM THE AUTHOR

I appreciate your time and attention, and I wish you well on your journey implementing functional medicine into your practice. I know even if you cannot execute it all, if you find a section of this or a particular system of interest, you can maximize patient's function and improve quality of life for many.

Minimal reductions in weight, addition of healthy fats in the diet, reduction of saturated fats, increased activity, and better glucose control could amount for drastic improvement in worldwide health.[89] Better health equates to less health-care costs and happier populations. AMA reports a 42 percent reduction in health-care expenditure with lifestyle modifications.[90]

In my opinion, physicians who care for patients for whom they can help feel better will suffer from burnout less than those treating symptoms and more symptoms without optimal health outcomes. By applying the basic functional medicine principles or detailed applications of the functional medicine matrix (if and when you are

---

[89] D. T. Jamison, J. G. Breman, A. R. Measham, et al., eds., *Disease Control Priorities in Developing Countries*, 2nd ed. Washington (DC): The International Bank for Reconstruction and Development / The World Bank; New York: Oxford University Press, 2006.

[90] Tamkeen Khan, Stavros Tsipas, and Gregory D. Wozniak, "Medical Care Expenditures for Individuals with Prediabetes: The Potential Cost Savings in Reducing the Risk of Developing Diabetes," *Population Health Management* (October 1, 2017), DOI: 10.1089/pop.2016.0134.

able), you can optimize biochemistry and support genetic variances, and if you too live the example of good self-care, you will restore your passion for your career choice, and your patients will more than appreciate your assistance!

APPENDIX A—MSQ

MSQ - MEDICAL SYMPTOM/TOXICITY QUESTIONNAIRE

NAME: _____ DATE: _____

The Toxicity and Symptom Screening Questionnaire identifies symptoms that help to identify the underlying causes of illness, and helps you track your progress over time. Rate each of the following symptoms based upon your health profile for the past 30 days. If you are taking after the first time, record your symptoms for the last 48 hours ONLY.

POINT SCALE
0 = Never or almost never have the symptom
1 = Occasionally have it, effect is not severe
2 = Occasionally have, effect is severe
3 = Frequently have it, effect is not severe
4 = Frequently have it, effect is severe

DIGESTIVE TRACT
___ Nausea or vomiting
___ Diarrhea
___ Constipation
___ Bloated feeling
___ Belching, or passing gas
___ Heartburn
___ Intestinal/Stomach pain
Total 0

EARS
___ Itchy ears Total
___ Earaches, ear infections
___ Drainage from ear
___ Ringing in ears, hearing loss
Total 0

EMOTIONS
___ Mood swings
___ Anxiety, fear or nervousness
___ Anger, irritability, or aggressiveness
___ Depression
Total 0

ENERGY/ACTIVITY
___ Fatigue, sluggishness
___ Apathy, lethargy
___ Hyperactivity
___ Restlessness
Total 0

EYES
___ Watery or itchy eyes
___ Swollen, reddened or sticky eyelids
___ Bags or dark circles under eyes
___ Blurred or tunnel vision (does not include near-or far-sightedness)
Total 0

HEAD
___ Headaches
___ Faintness
___ Dizziness
___ Insomnia
Total 0

HEART
___ Irregular or skipped heartbeat
___ Rapid or pounding heartbeat
___ Chest pain
Total 0

JOINTS/MUSCLES
___ Pain or aches in joints
___ Arthritis
___ Stiffness or limitation of movement
___ Pain or aches in muscles
___ Feeling of weakness or tiredness
Total 0

LUNGS
___ Chest congestion
___ Asthma, bronchitis
___ Shortness of breath
___ Difficult breathing
Total 0

MIND
___ Poor memory
___ Confusion, poor comprehension
___ Poor concentration
___ Poor physical coordination
___ Difficulty in making decisions
___ Stuttering or stammering
___ Slurred speech
___ Learning disabilities
Total 0

MOUTH/THROAT
___ Chronic coughing
___ Gagging, frequent need to clear throat
___ Sore throat, hoarseness, loss of voice
___ Swollen/discolored tongue, gum, lips
___ Canker sores
Total 0

NOSE
___ Stuffy nose
___ Sinus problems
___ Hay fever
___ Sneezing attacks
___ Excessive mucus formation
Total 0

SKIN
___ Acne
___ Hives, rashes, or dry skin
___ Hair loss
___ Flushing or hot flushes
___ Excessive sweating
Total 0

WEIGHT
___ Binge eating/drinking
___ Craving certain foods
___ Excessive weight
___ Compulsive eating
___ Water retention
___ Underweight
Total 0

OTHER
___ Frequent illness
___ Frequent or urgent urination
___ Genital itch or discharge
Total 0

GRAND TOTAL 0

KEY TO QUESTIONNAIRE
Add individual scores and total each group. Add each group scores and give a grand total.
• Optimal is less than 10   • Mild Toxicity: 10-50   • Moderate Toxicity: 50-100   • Severe Toxicity: over 100

MSQ appendix A

APPENDIX B

Y. F. Wang, J. F. Heng, J. Yan, and L. Dong, "Relationship between disease severity and thyroid function in Chinese patients with euthyroid sick syndrome," *Medicine* (Baltimore) 97(31)(2018): e11756.

ABSTRACT

Euthyroid sick syndrome (ESS) is commonly observed in various acute and chronic illness as risk factor for mortality in patients with severe diseases, with lower triiodothyronine (T3) and free triiodothyronine (fT3). To explore the relationship between disease severity and thyroid function in critically ill Chinese patients with ESS. A total of 51 patients admitted to intensive care unit were examined to determine acute physiology and chronic health assessment II (APACHE II) scores within 24 hours of admission; thyroid function tests (TSH, fT3, fT4, tT3, tT4) and rT3 levels were determined on the second day. Based on the test results, patients were divided into euthyroid (n=13), decreased fT3 or fT4 (n=17), and decreased TSH (n=21) groups. APACHE II scores and thyroid function were compared between the 3 groups. Furthermore, the relationship between the severity of disease and euthyroid sick syndrome was assessed. Out of 51 patients, 38 were men and 13 were women [mean age (± SD): 60.39 (± 19.32) years; range, 15-88 years]. APACHE II scores and rT3 levels were increased in all the 3 groups (P>.05). APACHE II scores showed a positive correlation with rT3 (P=.004, r=0.379). Critically ill Chinese patients with ESS have a poor health state. Higher rT3 values are associated with severe disease.

REGISTERED DIETICIANS

BeingBrigid.com—MS, RDN, LD, IFNCP—"graduate school professor and entrepreneur"

Fwdfuel.com—MS, RDN, CSSD, CLT, IFNCP—"Kylene specialized in athletic nutrition"

Tim Steen—ultra runner and RD with functional medicine nutrition specialty training, Master's student in dietetics, University of Arkansas

CONSOLIDATED REFERENCES

INTRODUCTION

Lee, J. Y., M. E. C. Abundo, and C. W. Lee, "Herbal Medicines with Antiviral Activity Against the Influenza Virus, a Systematic Review," *Am J Chin Med* 46(8)(2018): 1663–1700.

Li, Jiang-Hua, Zhi-Hui Wang, Xiao-Juan Zhu, Zhao-Hui Deng, Can-Xin Cai, Li-Qiang Qiu, Wei Chen, and Ya-Jun Lin, "Health Effects from Swimming Training in Chlorinated Pools and the Corresponding Metabolic Stress Pathways," *PLoS* 10(3)(March 5, 2015).

Bee Ling, Tan, Mohd Esa Norhaizanand, and Winnie-Pui-Pui Liew. "Nutrients and Oxidative Stress: Friend or Foe?" *Oxid Med Cell Longev* (2018), DOI:10.1155/2018/9719584.

Provenza, Frederick D.,[1*] Scott L. Kronberg,[2] and Pablo Gregorini.[3] "Is Grassfed Meat and Dairy Better for Human and Environmental Health?" *Front Nutr* 6(2019): 26. DOI:10.3389/fnut.2019.00026.

CHAPTER ONE

Lee, J. Y., M. E. C. Abundo, and C. W. Lee. "Herbal Medicines with Antiviral Activity Against the Influenza Virus, a Systematic Review." *Am J Chin Med* 46(8)(2018): 1663–1700.

Jiang-Hua, Li, Zhi-Hui Wang, Xiao-Juan Zhu, Zhao-Hui Deng, Can-Xin Cai, Li-Qiang Qiu, Wei Chen, and Ya-Jun Lin. "Health Effects from Swimming Training in Chlorinated Pools and the Corresponding Metabolic Stress Pathways." *PLoS* 10(3)(2015).

Beidelschies, Michelle, PhD[1], Marilyn Alejandro-Rodriguez, BSAS[1], Xinge Ji, MS[2], et al. "Association of the Functional Medicine Model of Care with Patient-Reported Health-Related Quality-of-Life Outcomes." *JAMA* 2(10)(2019): e1914017, DOI:10.1001.

Racine, A. D. "Providers and patients face-to-face: what is the time?" *Isr J Health Policy Res* 6(54)(2017), DOI:10.1186/s13584-017-0180-1.

Pirahanchi, Yasaman, and Ishwarlal Jialal. "Physiology, Thyroid Stimulating Hormone (TSH)," https://www.ncbi.nlm.nih.gov/books/NBK499850.

Becker, W. J. "The Diagnosis and Management of Chronic Migraine in Primary Care." *Headache* 57(9)(2017): 1471–1481..

Tlaskalová-Hogenová, H., L. Tucková, R. Stepánková, T. Hudcovic, L. Palová-Jelínková, and N. Y. "Involvement of innate immunity in the development of inflammatory and autoimmune diseases." *Ann Acad Sci* 1051(2005): 787–98, PMID: 16127016. DOI:10.1196/annals.1361.122.

CHAPTER TWO

Tuso, Philip J., MD. "Nutritional Update for Physicians: Plant-Based Diets." *Perm J* 17(2)(2013): 61–66, PMID: 23704846, PMCID: PMC3662288, DOI:10.7812/TPP/12-085.

Hussain, Joy, and Marc Cohen. "Clinical Effects of Regular Dry Sauna Bathing: A Systematic Review." *Evid Based Complement Alternat Med* 1857413(2018).

Laukkanen, Tanjaniina, Hassan Khan, Francesco Zaccardi, and Jari A. Laukkanen. "Association Between Sauna Bathing and Fatal Cardiovascular and All-Cause Mortality Events." *JAMA Internal Medicine* (2015), DOI:10.1001/jamainternmed.2014.8187.

Laukkanen, Tanjaniina, Setor Kunutsor, Jussi Kauhanen, and Jari Antero Laukkanen. "Sauna bathing is inversely associated with dementia and Alzheimer's disease in middle-aged Finnish men." *Age and Ageing* 46(2)(2017): 245–249.

Matsushita, K., A. Masuda, and C. Tei. "Efficacy of Infrared Sauna Therapy for Fibromyalgia." *Internal Medicine* 47(16)(2008): 1473–1476.

Mercola, Joseph. "How to Achieve Superior Detoxification and Health Benefits With Near-Infrared Light," Interview with Dr Brian Richards, www.mercola.com.

Shang-Ru Tsai, PhD, and Michael R Hamblin, PhD. "Biological effects and medical applications of infrared radiation." *J Photochem Photobiol B* 170(2017): 197–207. DOI:10.1016/j.jphotobiol.2017.04.014, PMCID: PMC5505738, NIHMSID: NIHMS870595, PMID: 28441605.

Vatansever, Fatma, and Michael R. Hamblin. "Far infrared radiation (FIR): its biological effects and medical applications." *Photonics Lasers Med* 4(2012): 255–266. DOI: 10.1515/plm-2012-0034, PMCID: PMC3699878, NIHMSID: NIHMS426504, PMID: 23833705.

"How LED Lighting May Compromise Your Health," https://globalpossibilities.org/how-led-lighting-may-compromise-your-health-3.

Tan, J., Y. Wang, Y. Xia, N. Zhang, X. Sun, T. Yu, and Lin. "Melatonin protects the esophageal epithelial barrier by suppressing the transcription, expression and activity of myosin light chain kinase through ERK1/2 signal transduction." *Cell Physiol Biochem* 34(6)(2014): 2117–2127. DOI: 10.1159/000369656.

Jialal, I., and U. Rajamani. "Endotoxemia of metabolic syndrome: a pivotal mediator of meta-inflammation." *Metab Syndr Relat Disord* 12(9)(2014): 454–456. DOI: 10.1089.

Hussain, Joy, and Marc Cohen. Clinical Effects of Regular Dry Sauna Bathing: A Systematic Review." *Evid Based Complement Alternat Med* (2018): 1857413. doi.org/10.1155/2018/1857413.

Laukkanen, Tanjaniina, Hassan Khan, Francesco Zaccardi, and Jari A. Laukkanen. "Association Between Sauna Bathing and Fatal Cardiovascular and All-Cause Mortality Events." *JAMA Internal Medicine* (2015). DOI: 10.1001/jamainternmed.2014.8187.

Tanjaniina, Laukkanen, Setor Kunutsor, Jussi Kauhanen, and Jari Antero Laukkanen. "Sauna bathing is inversely associated with dementia and Alzheimer's disease in middle-aged Finnish men." *Age and Ageing* 46(2)(2017): 245–249. doi.org/10.1093/ageing/afw212.

Matsushita, K., A. Masuda, and C. Tei. "Efficacy of Infrared Sauna Therapy for Fibromyalgia." 47(16)(2008): 1473–476.

Mercola, Joseph. "How to Achieve Superior Detoxification and Health Benefits With Near-Infrared Light." Interview with Dr. Brian Richards. Mercola.com.

Shang-Ru Tsai, PhD, and Michael R Hamblin, PhD. "Biological effects and medical applications of infrared radiation." *J Photochem Photobiol B* 170(2017): 197–207. PMCID: PMC5505738, NIHMSID: NIHMS870595, PMID: 28441605, DOI: 10.1016/j.jphotobiol.2017.04.014.

Vatansever, Fatma, and Michael R. Hamblin. "Far infrared radiation (FIR): its biological effects and medical applications." *Photonics Lasers Med* 4(2012): 255–266. DOI: 10.1515/plm-2012-0034, PMCID: PMC3699878, NIHMSID: NIHMS426504, PMID: 23833705.

Frazier, Thomas H., MD, John K. DiBaise, MD, and Craig J. McClain, MD. "Gut Microbiota, Intestinal Permeability, Obesity-Induced Inflammation, and Liver Injury." *Journal of Parenteral and Enteral Nutrition* 2011. DOI: 10.1177/0148607111413772.

Cani, Patrice D.,* Melania Osto, Lucie Geurts, and Amandine Everard. "Involvement of gut microbiota in the development of low-grade inflammation and type 2 diabetes associated with obesity." *Gut Microbes* 3(4)(2012): 279–288. PMCID: PMC3463487, PMID: 22572877, DOI: 10.4161/gmic.19625.

Escobedo G, E. López-Ortiz, and Torres-Castro. "Gut microbiota as a key player in triggering obesity, systemic inflammation and insulin resistance." *Rev Invest Clin* 66(5)(2014): 450–459. PMID: 25695388.

CHAPTER THREE

Taylor-Robinson, A. W., and R. S. Phillips. "B cells are required for the switch from Th1- to Th2-regulated immune responses to Plasmodium chabaudi infection." *Infect Immun* 62(6)(1994): 2490–2498. PMID: 8188374, PMCID:PMC186536.

Kizilbash, Sarah J., MD, Shelley P. Ahrens, RN, CNP, DNP, Barbara K. Bruce, PhD, Gisela Chelimsky, MD, et al., "Adolescent Fatigue, POTS, and Recovery: A Guide for Clinicians." *Curr Probl Pediatr Adolesc Health Care* 44(5)(2014): 108–133. PMID: 24819031, DOI: 10.1016/j.cppeds.2013.12.014.

Boone et al., "Mitochondrial dysfunction and the pathophysiology of Myalgic Encephalomyelitis/Chronic Fatigue Syndrome (ME/CFS)." *Int J Clin Exp Med* 5(3)(2012): 208–220. PMID: 22837795, PMCID: PMC3403556.

Unger, Elizabeth R., PhD, MD[1], Jin-Mann Sally Lin, PhD[1], Dana J. Brimmer, PhD, et al. "Chronic Fatigue Syndrome—Advancing Research and Clinical Education." *Weekly* (December 30, 2016)/65(5051): 1434–1438.

https://med.stanford.edu/news/all-news/2017/07/researchers-id-biomarkers-associated-withchronic-fatigue-syndrome.html.

Ahmetov, V. A., A. E. Naumov, A. Donnikov, E. S. Maciejewska-Karłowska, A. K. Kostryukova, and Larin. "*SOD2* gene polymorphism and muscle damage markers in elite athletes." *Free Radic Res* (2014): 948–955. DOI: 10.3109/10715762.2014.928410.

Yamano, E., M. Sugimoto, A. Hirayama, S. Kume, M. Yamato, G. Jin, and Y. Kataoka. "Index markers of chronic fatigue syndrome with dysfunction of TCA and urea cycles." *Scientific Reports 6* [34990](2016). https://doi.org/10.1038/srep34990.

Fischer, Alexandra, et al. "Association between genetic variants in the Coenzyme Q10 metabolism and Coenzyme Q10 status in humans." *BMC Res Notes* 4(2011): 245. DOI: 10.1186/1756-0500-4-245.

Williams, Luke R., Laura L. Quinn, Martin Rowe, and K. Jianmin Zuo. "Pathogenesis and Immunity-Induction of the Lytic Cycle Sensitizes Epstein-Barr Virus-Infected B Cells to NK Cell Killing That Is Counteracted by Virus-Mediated NK Cell Evasion Mechanisms in the Late Lytic Cycle." *Journal of Virology* (2015). DOI: 10.1128/JVI.01932-15.

Yao, QY, A. B. Rickinson, and M. A. Epstein. "A re-examination of the Epstein-Barr virus carrier state in healthy seropositive individuals." *Int J Cancer* 35(1985): 35–42. PMID: 2981780, DOI:10.1002/ijc.2910350107.

De Paschale M, Clerici Pierangelo. "Serological diagnosis of Epstein-Barr virus infection: Problems and Solutions." *World J Virol* 1(1)(2012): 31–43. DOI: 10.5501/wjv.v1.i1.31.

Liguori, Ilaria, Gennaro Russo, Francesco Curcio, Giulia Bulli, Luisa Aran, David Della-Morte, Gaetano Gargiulo, Gianluca Testa, Francesco Cacciatore, Domenico Bonaduce, and Pasquale Abete. "Oxidative stress, aging, and diseases." *Clin Interventional Aging* 13(2018): 757–772. DOI: 10.2147/CIA.S158513, PMCID: PMC5927356, PMID: 29731617

Micol, V.[1], N. Caturla, L. Pérez-Fons, V. Más, L. Pérez, and A. Estepa. "The olive leaf extract exhibits antiviral activity against viral haemorrhagic septicaemia rhabdovirus (VHSV)." *Antiviral Res* 66(2–3) (2005): 129–136. PMID: 15869811.

ABSTRACT

A commercial plant extract derived from olive tree leaf (Olea europaea) (LExt) and its major compound, oleuropein (Ole), inhibited the in vitro infectivity of the viral haemorrhagic septicaemia virus (VHSV), a salmonid rhabdovirus. Incubation of virus with LExt or Ole before infection reduced the viral infectivity to 10 and 30%, respectively. Furthermore, LExt drastically decreased VHSV titers and viral protein accumulation (virucidal effect) in a dose dependent manner when added to cell monolayers 36 h post-infection. On the other hand, both the LExt and Ole were able to inhibit cell-to-cell membrane fusion induced by VHSV in uninfected cells, suggesting interactions with viral envelope. Therefore, we propose that O. europaea could be used as a potential source of promising natural antivirals, which have demonstrated to lack impact on health and environment. In addition, Ole could be used to design other related antiviral agents.

CHAPTER FOUR

Barrett, E. M., D. G. I. Scott, N. J. Wiles, and D. P. M. Symmons. "The impact of rheumatoid arthritis on employment status in the early years of disease: a UK community-based study." *Rheumatology* 39(12) (2000): 1403–1409. https://doi.org/10.1093/rheumatology/39.12.1403.

Zegkos, Thomas, George Kitas, and Theodoros Dimitroulas. "Cardiovascular risk in rheumatoid arthritis: assessment, management and next steps." *Ther Adv Musculoskeletal Dis* 8(3)(2016): 86–101. DOI:10.1177/1759720X16643340 PMCID: PMC4872174

Charles-Schoeman, Christina, MD, MS. "Cardiovascular Disease and Rheumatoid Arthritis: An Update." *Curr Rheumatol Rep* 14(5)(2012): 455–462. DOI: 10.1007/s11926-012-0271-5, PMCID: PMC3436948, NIHMSID: NIHMS393529, PMID: 22791398.

Desai, Rishi J., MS PhD, Wesley Eddings, PhD, Katherine P. Liao, MD MPH, Daniel H. Solomon, MD, MPH, and Seoyoung C. Kim, MD, ScD, MSCE. "Disease modifying anti-rheumatic drug use and the risk of incident hyperlipidemia in patients with early rheumatoid arthritis: A retrospective cohort study." *Arthritis Care Res (Hoboken)* 67(4)(2015): 457–466. DOI: 10.1002/acr.22483, PMCID: PMC4751079, NIHMSID: NIHMS634440, PMID: 25302481.

Belkaid, Yasmine, and Timothy Hand. "Role of the Microbiota in Immunity and inflammation." Cell 157(1)(2014): 121–141. DOI: 10.1016/j.cell.2014.03.011, PMCID: PMC4056765, NIHMSID: NIHMS579635, PMID: 24679531.

Lazar, Veronica, Lia-Mara Ditu, Gratiela Gradisteanu Pircalabioru, Irina Gheorghe, Carmen Curutiu, Alina Maria Holban, Ariana Picu, Laura Petcu, and Mariana Carmen Chifiriuc. "Aspects of Gut Microbiota and Immune System Interactions in Infectious Diseases, Immunopathology, and Cancer." Front Immunol (August 15, 2018). https://doi.org/10.3389/fimmu.2018.01830.

Corthésy, Blaise. "Multi-Faceted Functions of Secretory IgA at Mucosal Surfaces." *Front Immunol* 4(2013): 185. DOI: 10.3389/fimmu.2013.00185, PMCID: PMC3709412, PMID: 23874333.

rheumatoidarthritis.org

Desai, MS PhD, Wesley Eddings, PhD, Katherine P. Liao, MD, MPH, Daniel H. Solomon, MD, MPH, and Seoyoung C. Kim, MD, ScD, MSCE, and J. Rishi. "Disease modifying anti-rheumatic drug use and the risk of incident hyperlipidemia in patients with early rheumatoid arthritis: A retrospective cohort study." *Arthritis Care Res (Hoboken)* 67(4) (2015): 457–466. DOI: 10.1002/acr.22483, PMCID: PMC4751079.

Corthésy, Blaise. "Multi-Faceted Functions of Secretory IgA at Mucosal Surfaces." Front Immunol 4 (2013): 185. DOI: 10.3389/fimmu.2013.00185, PMCID: PMC3709412, PMID: 23874333.

CHAPTER FIVE

de Benoist, Bruno, Maria Andersson, Bahi Takkouche, and Ines Egli. "Prevalence of iodine deficiency worldwide." *Lancet* (November 29, 2003). DOI: https://doi.org/10.1016/S0140-6736(03)14920-3.

Pingitore A., E. Galli, A. Barison, A. Iervasi, M. Scarlattini, D. Nucci, A. L'abbate, R. Mariotti, and G. Iervasi. "Acute effects of triiodothyronine (T3) replacement therapy in patients with chronic heart failure and low-T3 syndrome: a randomized, placebo-controlled study." *J Clin Endocrinol Metab* 93(4)(2008): 1351–1358. DOI: 10.1210/jc.2007-2210.

Ruiz-Núñez, Begoña, Rabab Tarasse, Emar F. Vogelaar, D. A. Janneke Dijck-Brouwer, and A. J. Frits. . "Higher Prevalence of 'Low T3 Syndrome' in Patients With Chronic Fatigue Syndrome: A Case–Control Study." *Frontiers of Endocrinology* 9(2018): 97. DOI: 10.3389/fendo.2018.00097, PMCID: PMC5869352, PMID: 29615976.

Park, E., J. Jung, O. Araki, et al. "Concurrent *TSHR* mutations and *DIO2* T92A polymorphism result in abnormal thyroid hormone metabolism." Sci Rep 8 (10090)(July 2018). DOI:10.1038/s41598-018-28480-0.

de Benoist, Bruno, Maria Andersson, Bahi Takkouche, and Ines Egli. "Prevalence of iodine deficiency worldwide." *Lancet* (November 29, 2003). DOI: https://doi.org/10.1016/S0140-6736(03)14920-3.

Pingitore, A., E. Galli, A. Barison, A. Iervasi, M. Scarlattini, D. Nucci, A. L'abbate, R. Mariotti, and G. Iervasi. "Acute effects of triiodothyronine (T3) replacement therapy in patients with chronic heart failure and low-T3 syndrome: a randomized, placebo-controlled study." *J Clin Endocrinol Metab* (4)(2008): 1351–1358. DOI: 10.1210/jc.2007-2210.

Nelson, J. C., and R. T. Tomei. "Direct determination of free thyroxin in undiluted serum by equilibrium dialysis/radioimmunoassay." *Clin Chem* 34(1988): 1737–1744. PMID: 3138040.

Wiersinga. "Therapy of Endocrine Disease: T4 + T3 combination therapy: is there a true effect?" *Eur J Endocrinol* 177(6)(2017): R287–R296. DOI:10.1530/EJE-17-0645.

Biondi, B., and D. S. Cooper. "The clinical significance of subclinical thyroid dysfunction." *Endocr Rev* 29(2008): 76–131. PMID:17991805, DOI:10.1210/er.2006-0043.

Cooper, D. S., and B. Biondi. "Subclinical thyroid disease." *Lancet* 379(2012): 1142–1154. DOI:10.1016/S0140-6736(11)60276-6.

Fernandes de Abreu, D. A., D. Eyles, and F. Féron. "Vitamin D, a neuro-immunomodulator: implications for neurodegenerative and autoimmune diseases." *Psychoneuroendocrinology* (December 1, 2009): S265–277. DOI:10.1016/j.psyneuen.2009.05.023.

Hoermann, R., J. E. M. Midgley, R. Larisch, and J. Dietrich. "Lessons from Randomised Clinical Trials for Triiodothyronine Treatment of Hypothyroidism: Have They Achieved Their Objectives?" *Thyroid Res* (July 16, 2018). DOI:10.1155/2018/3239197.

Chopra, Inder J. "Euthyroid Sick Syndrome: Is It a Misnomer?" *The Journal of Clinical Endocrinology & Metabolism* 82 (2)(1997): 329–334. https://doi.org/10.1210/jcem.82.2.3745.

Chopra, I. J. "An assessment of daily turnover and significance of thyroidal secretion of reverse T3 in man." *J Clin Invest* 58(1976): 32–40.

Nelson, J. C., and R.T. Tomei. "Direct determination of free thyroxin in undiluted serum by equilibrium dialysis/radioimmunoassay." *Clin Chem* 34(1988): 1737–1744. DOI: 10.1373.

Kaptein, E. M., W. J. Robinson, D. A. Grieb, and J. T. Nicoloff. "Peripheral serum thyroxine, triiodothyronine and reverse triodothyronine kinetics in the low thyroxine state of acute nonthyroidal illnesses. *J Clin Invest* 69(1982): 526–535.

Suda, A. K., C. S. Pittman, T. Shimizu, and J. B. Chambers Jr. "The production, and metabolism of 3,5,3'triiodothyronine and 3,3',5'-triiodothyronine in normal and fasting subjects." *J Clin Endocrinol Metab* 47(1978): 1311–1319.

Chopra, I. J., U. Chopra, S. R. Smith, M. Reza, and D. H. Solomon. "Reciprocal changes in serum concentrations of 3,3',5'-triiodothyronine (reverse T3) and 3,3',5-triiodothyronine (T3) in systemic illnesses." *J Clin Endocrinol Metab* 41(1975): 1043–1049. PMID:263351, DOI: 10.1210/jcem-47-6-1311.

Cardoso, B. A., and D. Rosenthal. "Thyroxine (T4) and triiodothyronine (T3) metabolism in normal subjects from Rio de Janeiro, Brazil." *Braz J Med Biol Res* 20(3–4)(1987): 419–423. PMID:3330463.

Wang, Y. F., J. F. Heng, J. Yan, and L. Dong. "Relationship between disease severity and thyroid function in Chinese patients with euthyroid sick syndrome." *Medicine* (Baltimore) 97(31)(2018): e11756.

Abstract: Euthyroid sick syndrome (ESS) is commonly observed in various acute and chronic illness as risk factor for mortality in patients with severe diseases, with lower triiodothyronine (T3) and free triiodothyronine (fT3).To explore the relationship between disease severity and thyroid function in critically ill Chinese patients with ESS.A total of 51 patients admitted to intensive care unit were examined to determine acute physiology and chronic health assessment II (APACHE II) scores within 24hours of admission; thyroid function tests (TSH, fT3, fT4, tT3, tT4) and rT3 levels were determined on the second day. Based on the test results, patients were divided into euthyroid (n=13), decreased fT3 or fT4 (n=17), and decreased TSH (n=21) groups. APACHE II scores and thyroid function were compared between the 3 groups. Furthermore, the relationship between the severity of disease and euthyroid sick syndrome was assessed. Out of 51 patients, 38 were men and 13 were women [mean age (± SD): 60.39 (± 19.32) years; range, 15-88 years]. APACHE II scores and rT3 levels were increased in all the 3 groups (P>.05). APACHE II scores showed a positive correlation with rT3 (P=.004, r=0.379). Critically ill Chinese patients with ESS have a poor health state. Higher rT3 values are associated with severe disease.

Gou, D. Y., W. Su, Y. C. Shao, and Y. L. Lu. "Euthyroid sick syndrome in trauma patients with severe inflammatory response syndrome." *Chin J Traumatol* 9(2)(2006): 115–117. PMID:16533439.

Alrefaie, Z., and H. Awad. "Effect of vitamin D3 on thyroid function and de-iodinase 2 expression in diabetic rats." *Arch Physiol Biochem* 121(5)(2015): 206–209. DOI:10.3109/13813455.2015.1107101.

CHAPTER SIX

Karras, S., E. Rapti, S. Matsoukas, and K. Kotsa. "Vitamin D in Fibromyalgia: A Causative or Confounding Biological Interplay?" *Nutrients* 8(6)(2016). PubMed #27271665.

Fernandes de Abreu, D. A., D. Eyles, and F. Féron. "Vitamin D, a neuro-immunomodulator: implications for neurodegenerative and autoimmune diseases." *Psychoneuroendocrinology* 34 (Suppl 1)(2009): S265–S277. DOI:10.1016.

Haidong, Zhu, Jigar Bhagatwala, Ying Huang, Norman K. Pollock, Samip Parikh, Anas Raed, Bernard Gutin, Gregory A. Harshfield, and Yanbin Dong. "Race/Ethnicity-Specific Association of Vitamin D and Global DNA Methylation: Cross-Sectional and Interventional Findings." *PLoS One* 11(4)(2016): e0152849. DOI:10.1371/journal.pone.0152849, PMCID: PMC4822838, PMID: 27049643.

Gallagher, J. Christopher, MD, MRCP. "Vitamin D and Aging." *Endocrinol Metab Clin North Am* 42(2)(2013): 319–332. DOI:10.1016/j.ecl.2013.02.004, PMCID: PMC3782116, NIHMSID: NIHMS46644, PMID: 23702404.

Schwartzman, M. S., and W. A. Franck. "Vitamin D toxicity complicating the treatment of senile, postmenopausal, and glucocorticoid-induced osteoporosis. Four case reports and a critical commentary on the use of vitamin D in these disorders." *Am J Med* 82(2)(1987): 224–230. PMID:3812514, DOI:10.1016/0002-9343(87)90060.

Wacker, Matthias, and Michael F. Holick. "A global perspective for health." *Dermatoendocrinol* 5(1)(2013): 51–108. PMCID:PMC3897598, PMID:24494042, DOI:10.4161/derm.24494.

Mullur, Rashmi, Yan-Yun Liu, and Gregory A. Brent. "Thyroid Hormone Regulation of Metabolism." *Physiol Rev* 94(2)(2014): 355–382. DOI:10.1152/physrev.00030.2013, PMCID:PMC4044302, PMID:24692351.

van Ballegooijen, Adriana J., Stefan Pilz, Andreas Tomaschitz, Martin R. Grübler, and Nicolas Verheyen. "The Synergistic Interplay between Vitamins D and K for Bone and Cardiovascular Health: A Narrative

Review." *Int J Endocrinol* (Sept. 12, 2017). DOI:10.1155/2017/7454376, PMCID:PMC5613455, PMID:29138634.

Karras, S., E. Rapti, S. Matsoukas, and K. Kotsa. "Vitamin D in Fibromyalgia: A Causative or Confounding Biological Interplay?" *Nutrients* 8(6)(2016). PubMed #27271665.

www.ingramcontent.com/pod-product-compliance
Lightning Source LLC
Chambersburg PA
CBHW020423220526
45464CB00002B/544